LIVING ON THE SPECTRUM

ANTHROPOLOGIES OF AMERICAN MEDICINE: CULTURE, POWER, AND PRACTICE

General Editors: Paul Brodwin, Michele Rivkin-Fish, and Susan Shaw

Transnational Reproduction: Race, Kinship, and Commercial Surrogacy in India
Daisy Deomampo

Unequal Coverage: The Experience of Health Care Reform in the United States
Edited by Jessica Mulligan and Heide Castañeda

Inequalities of Aging: Paradoxes of Independence in American Home Care
Elana D. Buch

The New American Servitude: African Home Care Workers in the United States
Cati Coe

Racism and Reproductive Justice: Black Mothers, Premature Birth, and the NICU
Dána-Ain Davis

Living on the Spectrum: Autism and Youth in Community
Elizabeth Fein

Living on the Spectrum

Autism and Youth in Community

Elizabeth Fein

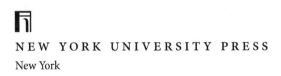

NEW YORK UNIVERSITY PRESS

New York

NEW YORK UNIVERSITY PRESS
New York
www.nyupress.org

References to Internet websites (URLs) were accurate at the time of writing. Neither the author nor New York University Press is responsible for URLs that may have expired or changed since the manuscript was prepared.

Library of Congress Cataloging-in-Publication Data
Names: Fein, Elizabeth, author.
Title: Living on the spectrum : autism and youth in community / Elizabeth Fein.
Description: New York : New York University Press, [2020] | Series: Anthropologies of American medicine | Includes bibliographical references and index.
Identifiers: LCCN 2019038485 | ISBN 9781479864355 (cloth) | ISBN 9781479889068 (paperback) | ISBN 9781479873005 (ebook) | ISBN 9781479848164 (ebook)
Subjects: LCSH: Autistic youth—United States—Attitudes. | Autistic youth—United States—Social conditions. | Youth with autism spectrum disorders—Education—United States.
Classification: LCC RC553.A88 F44 2020 | DDC 362.19685/882—dc23
LC record available at https://lccn.loc.gov/2019038485

New York University Press books are printed on acid-free paper, and their binding materials are chosen for strength and durability. We strive to use environmentally responsible suppliers and materials to the greatest extent possible in publishing our books.

Manufactured in the United States of America

10 9 8 7 6 5 4 3 2 1

Also available as an ebook

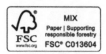

CONTENTS

CONTENTS

Introduction

Autism is like this.

It's like someone sneaks into your house, in the middle of the night, and takes your precious baby's mind, and personality—and leaves their bewildered body behind.
—Cure Autism Now, "Kidnapped"

Autism is a way of being. It is pervasive; it colors every experience, every sensation, perception, thought, emotion, and encounter, every aspect of existence. It is not possible to separate the autism from the person. . . .

Therefore, when parents say, I wish my child did not have autism, what they're really saying is, I wish the autistic child I have did not exist, and I had a different (non-autistic) child instead. Read that again. This is what we hear when you mourn over our existence. This is what we hear when you pray for a cure. This is what we know, when you tell us of your fondest hopes and dreams for us: that your greatest wish is that one day we will cease to be, and strangers you can love will move in behind our faces.
—Jim Sinclair, "Don't Mourn for Us" (1993, para. 5–7)

ELIZABETH: So you were saying that you heard this thing [on the news], that this woman was saying that autism was a disease?
ANDREW: Yeah, that really—that really set me off.
ELIZABETH: When was that?
ANDREW: A couple years ago. I really wanted to call up the person on live TV. That would have felt so good. But I couldn't find the number.
ELIZABETH: What would you have said if you could get hold of her?
ANDREW: I would've just started cursin' at her, sayin', you know, autism is not a disease, it's a developmental disability. Research it, why don't you. I wanted to point that out. Tell her: do some research.
ELIZABETH: Why do you think it was so important to you, like, that she got—
ANDREW: 'Cause she's making it sound like we're a bunch of diseased people, that we're diseased.
—Interview with Andrew Yollen, 17, diagnosed with Asperger's syndrome

Autism is a deeply contested condition. Sometimes, people talk about it as a public health crisis, an invading enemy to be identified and eliminated. Sometimes, people talk about it as a fundamental and valued aspect of personhood and identity, something to be protected rather than something to protect against. As autism rose to its extraordinary state of prominence over the past several decades, these two ways of talking about autism—and the conflicts between them—dominated a great deal of the public conversation.

For Andrew, 17 and diagnosed with Asperger's syndrome—a condition on the "autism spectrum"—these definitional battles over autism matter. As he tells us here, representations of autism affect his own sense of who he is and his sense of how others see him. But Andrew is telling us other things, as well. These conflicts, he wants us to know, are embedded in other distinctions, between *disease* and *developmental disability*. These distinctions are grounded in particular approaches to scientific practice that are accessible to the attentive layperson (*do some research!*), shaping his self-concept through their particular contours. And these distinctions, he tells us, matter for more than just Andrew himself. He is upset because the person on the news made it sound like *we're a bunch of diseased people*. He is not merely an *I*, a child alone in a room breached by an inhuman kidnapper. He is part of a *we*.

Once considered a rare and inevitably debilitating disorder, autism is now said by the Centers for Disease Control and Prevention to affect 1 out of every 59 children in the United States, in a wide variety of ways, across a spectrum of severity ranging from profoundly to mildly disabling (Baio et al., 2018). Driven by the advocacy of networks of families affected by autism, in collaboration with deeply committed groups of researchers, many resources have been allocated to understanding the biological basis of autism, in the hopes of finding better means to treat, prevent or cure it. At the same time, a growing movement of individuals on the autism spectrum, often referred to as (part of) the *neurodiversity movement*, argue that autism is instead a natural and valuable aspect of human diversity, a cultural identity calling for accommodation rather than prevention. A cure for autism would thus be not a mercy but a genocidal suppression of difference, equivalent to "curing" someone's race, gender, or sexual orientation.

These different positions—the notion of autism as a disease to be cured and the notion of autism as an identity to be respected—are often depicted within public discourse as being radically incompatible. But in practice, their coexistence is far more complex. Organizations seeking a cure or a means of prevention for autism increasingly draw on autism-positive, inclusive rhetoric to celebrate the appealing qualities of autistic people, while striving to distinguish these from the kind of problematic qualities that can remain comfortably within a cure-oriented medical paradigm. Discourses rooted in autistic self-advocacy and the celebration of neurodiversity are still intertwined with the assumptions of the medical paradigms within which they originated, in intricate and subtle ways. And people living with autism spectrum diagnoses must find ways to live under both of these descriptions, integrating these seemingly irreconcilable discourses in the business of their daily lives.

Watching these controversies unfold, I became curious about how they were affecting the rapidly expanding cohort of young people coming of age with an autism spectrum diagnosis. How were these youth reconciling these divergent sets of ideas about autism, the self, and the relationship between, in the context of their own developing identities? While these controversies have been very visible in spaces of public advocacy and representation (in the media, on blogs and websites, at conferences), there has been less sustained ethnographic exploration of these issues as they relate to the experiences of people who do not identify as authors, or advocates, or activists.[1] This book explores the ways that people directly affected by autism spectrum conditions—people with autism spectrum diagnoses, their families, and the practitioners who work with them—negotiate the meanings of this contested condition, in consequential ways, in the spaces where they live, learn, love, work, and play in their everyday lives. The research takes place on the East Coast of the United States, and I focus on those on the edges of the expanding autism spectrum—those, like Andrew, with conditions that were once called "Asperger's syndrome" or "high-functioning autism" or "pervasive developmental disorder, not otherwise specified" [PDD-NOS] —who are caught up in its broadening purview.

Much of the research on autism has been conducted in laboratories with individual research participants or in contexts where people on the autism spectrum represent a small and problematized minority among nonautistic people—trends that risk essentializing the stereotype of people with autism as fundamentally estranged from sociality, by nature at odd angles with shared culture. This book takes a different approach: It is based on ethnographic fieldwork in communities where people on the autism spectrum come together. Such spaces tend to assemble people who are affected by autism in a variety of ways: people who have the diagnosis, people who have interests in common with people who have the diagnosis, family members, professionals who have chosen to dedicate much of their professional lives to autism, and others as well. In such spaces, amidst the various propensities that get aggregated under and around the "autism concept" (Cascio, 2018), we can begin to trace some forms and manifestations of what could be called autistic culture.

This book chronicles the ways in which youth on the autism spectrum make sense of life under the description of autism. But the description under which they are living is not singular but multiple, not stable but shifting. As a developmental disability, autism is often defined in contrast to mental illnesses; it is assumed to be fixed, lifelong, and innate, whereas mental illness is assumed to be more fluid and transient. This distinction, however, is being unsettled through a paradigm shift in psychiatric diagnosis—what I talk about as a "neurodevelopmental turn"—away from an understanding of mental illnesses as discrete disease categories and toward the assessment and remediation of universally shared human capacities for perception, memory, attention, self-regulation, and learning. Construing mental disorders as neurodevelopmental produces diagnostic states that are experienced differently from those produced through its predecessor, the categorical approach to diagnosis that developed in and dominated the end of the 20th century. Conditions delineated through the "neurodevelopmental turn" are fundamentally intertwined with our sense of who we are, and with the world that surrounds us—how we learn, how we remember, how we attend, how we love. In some cases, they bring a complex package of benefits and drawbacks. Such neurodevelopmental conditions coexist uneasily with older approaches, from the previous psychiatric paradigm, within which disorders are defined more like pathogens rather than packages: as diseases to be eradicated, negative and separable and located exclusively within our bodies.

Through a process I call "divided medicalization," the former get misrepresented as the latter: Complex, multivalent neurodevelopmental conditions are produced and then reduced to fit within a preexisting, disease-oriented clinical paradigm. Through this process of expansion and constriction of diagnostic categories, phenomena that play out between the individual and the environment are *individualized*: Their social and sensory dimensions get mapped back onto the individual as the locus of explanation and site of intervention. Aspects of experience that transcend the bounds of the physical body—the connections between our selves and our social partners, between our senses and the things being sensed, between our attention and the material to which we attend, and so forth—are thus occluded, rendered invisible. This individualizing process of expansion and constriction perpetuates a severing of the self from its surroundings. What lies outside our skin is construed as irrelevant, or even antithetical, to who we are. In talking with families affected by autism spectrum conditions, I saw how this conceptualization of the self—the idea that we are defined entirely by our particular internal qualities, not by anything that exists beyond our bodies—undergirds the intractability of ethical conflicts over prevention and cure.

Notions of the self as sharply bounded and separate from a threatening outside world underlie medical conceptualizations of autism—whether autism is conceived of as an invading pathogen or as a hardwired neurogenetic identity that is destroyed if it is altered. Neither approach, however, is sufficient for capturing the full experience of youth on the autism spectrum. Instead, these youth look outside of medicine to find a shared language, articulating discontinuous and disconcertingly permeable identities through a shared folk mythology drawn from multimedia speculative fictions of mutation, possession, and hybridity. In doing so, these youth also formulate possibilities for a different way of being, one that is open to the surrounding environment in ways both dangerous and exciting. Through attending to their shared social practices, organized around the care and maintenance of locally interconnected systems, we can gain some insight into how to mitigate the loneliness and isolation that too often accompanies autistic difference, by intervening at the troubled intersection between the individual and their social surroundings. That space of intersection, I argue, is where autism happens.

According to the fifth edition of the *Diagnostic and Statistical Manual of Mental Disorders* (*DSM-5*; American Psychiatric Association, 2013), autism spectrum disorder is defined by the following symptoms, present from very early in life and causing clinically significant impairment:

> A. Persistent deficits in social communication and social interaction across multiple contexts, as manifested by: deficits in social-emotional reciprocity; deficits in nonverbal communicative behaviors used for social interaction; and deficits in developing, maintaining, and understanding relationships,

and

> B. Restricted, repetitive patterns of behavior, interests, or activities, as manifested by two or more of the following: stereotyped or repetitive motor movements, use of objects, or speech; insistence on sameness, inflexible adherence to routines or ritualized patterns of verbal or nonverbal behavior; highly restricted, fixated interests that are abnormal in intensity or focus; and/or hyper- or hyporeactivity to sensory input or unusual interest in sensory aspects of the environment.[2]

Autism is therefore an inherently paradoxical condition: a social disorder of the individual, a disorder of aloneness that can never be enacted alone. The word *autism* comes from the Greek *autos*, for *self*. But other people (social interlocutors, potential relational partners, co-participants in social failure), and other things (interests, routines, activities, objects, stimuli), are always a constitutive component of autism. When it comes to reciprocity, the formation or failure of relationships, or successful or unsuccessful communication, it takes (at least) two to tango. As for restricted interests, nobody is born into this world obsessed with Thomas the Tank Engine; the interest emerges through exposure to the content. One cannot be autistic in a vacuum. The kind of insular aloneness that the term *autism* has come to represent is contradicted by its very criteria.

This book aims to explore the origins and implications of this paradox: How does such an irreducibly social, cultural, and interpersonal phenomenon as autism come to connote the absence of sociality, relationality, and interpersonal significance? What kind of cultural meaning-work gets done through this transformation? In doing so, this book also explores the ground on which much of this work takes place: the contested terrain of the human brain.

Looping the Neuro

The ways in which we come to associate our sense of personhood, personality, and identity with our brains—and, in particular, our brains as they are known through scientific expertise, driven by particular techniques for abstraction, visualization, assessment, diagnosis, and intervention—has become a thriving topic of social scientific inquiry. How did we come to be so thoroughly identified with our brains and our brains alone—over and instead of other potential determinants (the rest of our bodies, our social relations, our place in a divine order, etc.)? What are the consequences of becoming such a "cerebral subject" (Ortega, 2009; Ortega & Vidal, 2007; Vidal & Ortega, 2017)? Many (e.g., see Martin, 2004) raise concerns about the hegemony of *neuro-reductionism*. Others, skeptics of all the *neuro-hype* (e.g., Satel, Marshall, Aslinger, & Lilienfield, 2013), are worried less about the impact of neuroscientific promises come true than about their expense and their lack of feasibility. These questions are often debated with a great deal of passion and theoretical insightfulness but without the empirical data that would allow us to see how particular strands of neuroscientific discourse are taken up by particular people with particular cognitive styles in particular contexts and mobilized to particular ends. This book aims to add something missing from many of these accounts: a sustained empirical engagement with the ways in which neuro-discourses are adopted or rejected, amplified or silenced, interpreted and enacted, mobilized and transformed, in contexts of everyday life. Much of the most influential theoretical work has focused on publicly circulating discourses and less on ethnographic study of how this circulation happens. This book, on the other hand, takes place in the spaces where the neuro is lived.

In such spaces, these discourses are transformed by the people who live them. Subjectivity is shaped by neuro-discourse, but neuro-discourses are also shaped by the subjects assembled under their descriptors. The philosopher Ian Hacking (1995) uses the phrase "the looping effect of human kinds" to describe the ways that living under a social scientific classification changes people—their self-concept, their behavior, even their biological makeup—in ways that then lead to changes to the classification itself, thus creating an ongoing feedback loop. This process applies to a wide variety of perceived human types, from "breast cancer survivor" to "child abuser." People react to the ways in which they are classified—sometimes living up to their labels, sometimes seeking to prove them wrong. Meanwhile, the experience of classification changes the people being classified such that they are not the same as they were before. Diagnoses provide access to new experiences: treatments, accommodations, group memberships, stigma, shame, pride. The people gathered under a diagnostic umbrella look around and see each other, and from that, they learn something about themselves; perhaps they form alliances, or perhaps they try to push each other out from under the umbrella. As the people change, the meaning of the word describing those people changes as well. For example, after several decades of work by people with what was once called "atypical autism" and their families to advocate for the inclusion and consideration of people with milder forms of autism under the spectrum umbrella, *autism* is no longer a word assumed to describe a severe and significant developmental delay. Now, a National Council on Severe Autism is being formed by parents increasingly concerned that it is the needs of people with what is sometimes called "classic autism," on "the severe end of the spectrum," that are currently being left out of conversations about autism (Opar, 2019). (This, I am uncomfortably aware, is a problem to which this book, which began as a research project on "Asperger's syndrome" and has now become a book about "the autism spectrum," could be said to contribute.) The word *autism* describes something very different than it once did. Types of people, Hacking (2007) observes, are thus "moving targets." To study this process, Hacking (2004) suggests, we need to work across disciplinary boundaries between levels of analysis, paying attention to both large-scale social and historical forces and the nuances of face-to-face interaction.

Autistic Presence

At least in the case of autism, I would argue, we need to consider another level, as well: the particularities of neurodevelopmental conditions themselves as shifting assemblages of cognitive, experiential, sensory, and interpretive processes. While an increasingly rich and varied body of work takes up the issue of culture and its influence on neurodevelopment (e.g., Brezis et al., 2016; Grinker, 2007; Ochs, Solomon, & Sterponi, 2005), this book thus seeks to add a deeper awareness of the ways in which patterned neurodevelopmental variation shapes social, cultural, and biopolitical processes. To give an example, when it comes to looping effects, a type such as "autism" functions differently from a type such as "breast cancer survivor." The autism diagnosis brings together people who share a particular interpretive style which often includes an intense interest in structured systems, such as those that produce social scientific classifications. In the case of autism, affinities between the cognitive style being scientifically classified and the processes of scientific classification itself result in the looping process being amplified such that people on the autism spectrum come to exemplify certain kinds of science. Understanding the process through which autism has come to its extraordinary state of prevalence and prominence therefore requires an understanding of aggregated patterns of cognitive, affective, and interpretive styles and their consequences for social processes.

Stuart Murray, a professor of contemporary literature and film who has written extensively on representations of autism, emphasizes the importance of attending to autistic *presence* instead of the metaphors of absence that characterize much of the discourse surrounding autism. "To extract autism," he writes, "from such an association—to properly look for its presence—is a process that requires an understanding of its formations that precede . . . public metaphors" (Murray, 2008, p. 28). Attending to autistic presence invites us to attend also to dimensions often excluded from representations of autism, such as pleasure, creativity, and humor (and sometimes also, I argue, meaningful rage, pain, and sorrow). It invites us to attend to lines of continuity between phenomena (behaviors, experiences, people, situations) that have been explicitly labeled with autism and those that have not. And it invites us into a flirtation with the risk of reifying biological difference. In what follows, I take seriously the notion that our physical bodies give rise to variations in our perceptions and interpretations, and that those variations are patterned in some regular ways. To quote autistic author Nick Walker (2014, para. 6), however, treating the "diversity of human brains and minds—the infinite variation in neurocognitive functioning within our species" as a "biological fact" does not prevent us from grappling with its varied social and political manifestations and meanings. Nor does a recognition that there are patterns of correlation between certain cognitive and interpretive styles—some of which get identified as pathological, some of which get identified as beneficial, and some of which occupy a vast and shifting gray area between. Discussions of autism that treat it as if it were the same as any other condition that is similar along some foregrounded axis (as analogous to other chronic illnesses or other forms of stigmatized difference or other grounds for biosocial group formation) contribute in some ways to the erasure of autistic presence. Listening to the patterns that get aggregated under autism diagnoses allows us instead to more fully recognize their social and moral implications.

Clinical Ethnography

I do so, here, through an approach known as *clinical ethnography*. Clinical ethnography works at the intersection of personhood and social world, illuminating the inextricability of domains associated with psychology and those associated with the anthropological study of culture. The phrase itself carries multiple sets of meanings. It can mean simply an ethnography of the clinic, an anthropological study of sites of distress and healing within particular practical and epistemological contexts; in this usage, the phrase is most often applied to ethnographies of psychiatric practice. But "clinical ethnography" can also mean an ethnography that is informed by clinical modes of engagement, interpretation, and inference, carried out by those with training in these modalities—in my case, having trained as a clinical psychologist.[3] My mode of observation is itself clinical, the lenses through which I view the world honed through training in both psychodynamic psychotherapy and neurodevelopmental assessment.

I understand clinical ethnography to be ethnography both *of* and *through* clinical traditions: bodies of culture-specific knowledge about how to perceive, engage with, assess, and transform the subjectivities of others. This book, for example, is an ethnographic study of neuropsychology as a practice; it also applies neuropsychological theories as an analytical lens on sociocultural processes. When we are studying aspects of our own professional communities, as I do here, clinical ethnography can be profoundly and disconcertingly reflexive, as the tools through which we do our work constitute both a process of analysis and its object. In my research and practice, I turn a critical eye toward the clinical traditions and tools of my own society while I also apply them in settings of care with people urgently seeking my help; the ongoing tension has produced in me a sort of uncomfortable, curious stance toward my own ways of knowing. If this book has been able to hold a space for multiplicity and ambivalence over singularity and polarization, as I have aimed here to do in my approach to some pretty divisive topics, it is, in large part, due to this way of inhabiting truths.

As Good et al. (1985) have observed, clinical ethnography is grounded in psychological traditions that foreground "the centrality of interpretation, the importance of studying the relation between public symbols, discourse, and personal meanings, and the theoretical and clinical importance of investigating the 'objectivity' of the analyst or observer in clinical encounters" (p. 193). Clinical ethnographers work with the kind of phenomena that, in many societies, are considered to be inner or internal, including those that may not be articulated explicitly in language or even present in conscious awareness. We therefore engage in processes of interpretation and inference from which our own inner lives and personal histories are inextricable. As a psychotherapist, I have learned to cultivate a careful awareness around what I myself bring to my attempts to understand the worlds of others, including my ethnographic work.

Autism is a condition that lives in the relational borderlands between self and other, subject and object, person and world. It takes form within our closest and most intimate personal ties, in the spaces where people who care for each other struggle to connect with each other, in the deep human yearning to share experience across difference and to be heard, recognized, and understood. Many of the people who have helped develop the concept of autism as it now exists—as researchers, therapists, self-advocates, activists, or in other roles—have experienced autism within such personal contexts and connections, and the nature of these histories have shaped the contours of what autism has become. My own history is no exception. Like others, I was initially drawn into an involvement with the autism spectrum through the experiences of someone I love.

Quiet Hands, Loud Hands

I first met A when he came along to a movie with a group of my friends. I remember a tall, blond fellow hanging out at the fringes, aloof, speaking only to offer cryptic commentary on the proceedings. *Who the hell does he think he is*, I recall thinking crossly, unimpressed. The next time I saw him was at a New Year's Eve party, the last night of 1998. He was standing in the corner of the host's living room, wrapped up in a long black overcoat and black gloves, unmoving and silent. Someone had decorated him with a string of Christmas lights. Later that evening, I found him sitting under a table brooding about the apocalyptic potential of the Y2K bug,[4] due to hit a year later. I ducked under there to join him. We spent the rest of that night talking and woke up, the first day of the last year of the millennium, wrapped in each other's arms. It was the beginning of a long love affair and a deep friendship. It was also the beginning of my awareness of Asperger's syndrome, sometime later, when his mother sent him a copy of Tony Attwood's (1997) *Asperger's Syndrome: A Guide for Parents and Professionals* as a sort of gentle hint. Nonplussed, he read a few sections to me over the phone. I was fascinated at the refraction of what I immediately recognized as a well-known folk category—the nerd, socially awkward, physically clumsy, and obsessed with arcane topics— into a medical diagnosis. I started going to talks about Asperger's at the hospital where I was working as an administrative assistant as I prepared to go to grad school, and took it up as my topic when I got there.

To me, the lens of the *neuro* therefore feels significant but not sufficient for framing a discussion of autism—a condition that plays out through whole bodies, in all their pluripotent possibilities. While brains, with their affordances both extensive and encapsulated, have become a predominant organizing metaphor for both autism and the self, other kinds of stories about autism center not in the brain, but in the hands. *Loud Hands* (Bascom, 2012), the title of an anthology published by the

Autistic Self-Advocacy Network, has more broadly become a rallying cry for the autistic self-advocacy movement, both a description of the stimming, flapping hand movements that are a fundamental aspect of autistic bodily experience and expression and a refusal of the demand for "quiet hands" that behavior therapists often use to keep them still. Autism is not only absence but also presence; autism is not only silence but also song. Have you ever seen Gary Numan perform live? I did, just last night. Gary Numan is a musician who has been quite public about his diagnosis of Asperger's syndrome. He writes songs about profound alienation and technological mediation, and over the course of a 40-year career has gone from being famous for his stiff and robotic stage presence to being a mesmerizing, kinetic live performer. His hands are everywhere—twisting, shaking, gesturing, exploring the air, slicing through the flashing lights, punctuating the stark rhythms. Hands hold; they communicate; they apprehend; they are sites of violence and intimacy. As phenomenologist philosopher Maurice Merleau-Ponty (1965) points out, hands exemplify the inevitable simultaneity of touching and being touched, which is, in many ways, what this book tries to be about. But this book is also about how large things get carved down into smaller ones and stories of shared interpersonal worlds become stories of bounded individual selves—a process that is deeply connected to our historically situated and shifting conceptions of the mind and brain.

Histories of Autism

As linguistic anthropologist Olga Solomon (2010) has observed, histories of autism often begin with an origin story that has become canonical, taking on mythic proportions; it is a story that foregrounds the work of single pioneers rather than the sociohistorical context that made their discoveries thinkable. Autism, the story begins, was discovered and named almost simultaneously in two different places by two different doctors. In 1943, Leo Kanner published a paper called "Autistic Disorders of Affective Contact," giving a detailed description of the "fascinating peculiarities" of a group of children he had seen in his practice. Kanner described these children as detached and inaccessible, preoccupied with repetitive behaviors whose meaning could not be shared with others. Meanwhile, in Vienna, pediatrician Hans Asperger (1944) was also identifying a "highly recognizable type of child" whose distinctive behaviors he, too, used the word *autistic* to describe. The children Asperger described, however, were more likely to be verbal, often highly so, perseverating endlessly on their topics of interest. To protect the children in his practice from the threat of extermination by the Nazi regime then in power, the story goes, Asperger emphasized their intellectual gifts and their potential to contribute to society. Kanner's understanding of autism—and his observation that the parents of these children, too, often appeared chilly and removed—was widely adopted throughout the second half of the 20th century, leading to a conception of autism as a profoundly impairing disorder and a misconception that it was caused by aloof parenting. Meanwhile, Asperger's work languished in obscurity until the 1980s, when clinician Lorna Wing translated it into English, taking up the term *Asperger's syndrome* to describe children she saw in her practice, who displayed the social detachment and repetitive behaviors associated with autism but who displayed normal or even extraordinary intellectual and language ability. Her work, along with others who began to investigate and treat Asperger's syndrome, drove the expansion of autism from a diagnostic descriptor of severe psychopathology to a spectrum with varied and diverse manifestations. In 1994, Asperger's disorder was added to the *DSM-IV* (American Psychiatric Association, 1994) as one of the five "pervasive developmental disorders" that make up the autism spectrum. In 2013, with the *DSM-5*, the American Psychiatric Association removed it, as these individual categories were rolled into one single "autism spectrum disorder."

Over the past several decades, the number of people diagnosed with autism spectrum conditions has risen sharply, with prevalence estimates rising from fewer than 5 per 10,000 in studies published in the 1980s to 1 in 59 today (Baio et al., 2018; Burd, Fisher, & Kerbeshian, 1987; Matson & Kozlowski, 2011; Ritvo et al., 1989). This rise has led to widespread concern about the emerging "autism epidemic," with some attempting to identify some pathogenic influence—most notoriously, but not exclusively, vaccination—that can explain and potentially mitigate it (e.g., Blaxill, 2004; Herbert, 2008). Others, however, have argued that the rise in autism's prevalence can be explained by changes in diagnostic classification criteria and the broader infrastructures in which they are embedded (Gernsbacher, Dawson, & Hill Goldsmith, 2005; Grinker, 2007).

This high-stakes debate has charged controversies over the ontological status and meaning of autism.

In its focus on individual people and the seemingly remarkable co-incidence of their simultaneous discoveries, the mythic origin story of autism downplays the many factors—from psychiatric reform and dein-stitutionalization to the increasing reliance on technological metaphors for the brain—within which autism in its current form is even conceiv-able. A number of recent historical accounts have sought to recontex-tualize autism within these broader milieux (Cascio, Costa Andrada, & Bezerra, 2018; Eyal, Hart, Oncluer, Oren, & Rossi, 2010; Lima, Feldman, Evans, & Block, 2018; Nadesan, 2005; Silberman, 2015).[5] Even the story of Hans Asperger as the savior of his "little scientists" has been challenged by recently unearthed records suggesting that he may simultaneously have been complicit in the consignment of those more severely impaired to murder at the hands of the Nazis. Furthermore, the very articula-tion of autism as a social psychopathology of absent fellow-feeling took form under the Nazi demand for assimilation and for compliance that is motivated by a sincere desire to conform to the group (Czech, 2018; Sheffer, 2018). From its very inception, these findings suggest, controver-sies about autism—its meaning and boundaries, its ability to expansively tie together a wide range of human capacities and vulnerabilities—have been bound up in the complex imbrications of healing and violence that emerge out of attempts to create not only healthy individuals but also healthy societies. When certain ways of being are considered outside of sociality, they are more likely to be considered outside of the protection, care, and respect afforded to human life.

In what follows, I try instead to consider neurocognitive variation, including that which is currently being assembled under the autism di-agnosis, as a constitutive aspect of shared social and cultural worlds. In the introduction to their volume *Schizophrenia, Culture and Subjectivity: The Edge of Experience*, psychological anthropologist Janis Hunter Jen-kins and psychiatrist and anthropologist Robert John Barrett (2004) lay out a set of orientation points for how to foreground culture and subjec-tivity in the study of conditions, such as schizophrenia, that are "situated at the margins of culture, at the very edge of meaningful experience" (p. 5). They suggest that we orient toward lived experience by work-ing with concepts and terms that are familiar to our participants rather than relying on experience-distant professional abstractions, emphasize the "active engagement of subjects in processes of cultural construction" rather than depicting subjects as passively shaped by a fixed and stable cultural system, and attend to "the irrepressibility of subjectivity as embedded in intersubjectively created realms of meaning and significance . . . as a bridge between individual experience and social reality" (pp. 8–9)—even, and especially, when considering people whose condition is mistakenly thought to block them from authentic participation in intersubjective life. These principles have guided the development and writing of this book.

About the Research

To research this book, I spent 2 years conducting ethnographic participant-observation—immersing myself in community life and activity—at a variety of sites where the meanings of autism spectrum conditions were being consequentially negotiated and put into practice. I focused on sites and programs serving those at the expanding edges of the autism spectrum. The project originally focused on Asperger's syndrome, and in many ways, the Asperger's phenomenon—certain kinds of struggles with sociality and a tendency toward certain forms of restriction and repetitiveness, reminiscent of severe autism but without language disorder or cognitive impairment—is still at the center of this book. However, while doing this work, I also came to understand that there is no clear dividing line between Asperger's syndrome and other autism spectrum conditions, and that most communities bringing together people with Asperger's include those with other related diagnoses—"high-functioning" autism, PDD-NOS, and so on—as well. The presumed dividing lines between diagnostic categories are messy in this book as they are in real life, and a lot of my work takes place amid the mess.

My fieldwork was divided between a rural area, which I call Brookfield, and a nearby city, which I call Park City, both on the East Coast of the United States. I spent time in two public and two private school classrooms, a community center and affiliated summer camp, a series of support groups, an after-school program, a clinic housed in a medical school, a research lab testing pharmaceutical treatments, and a series of local and national conferences, all serving people with Asperger's syndrome and related autism spectrum conditions. I also went to birthday parties, hung out informally with families, bowled with a bowling league, and ran focus groups at a science-fiction convention. During this time, I was taking field notes—jotting down notes as things were going on during the day and then typing them up for several hours each evening, often in a great deal of detail. Descriptions of events, and conversations not part of a recorded interview, have been reconstructed from these notes.

I also interviewed participants in these communities, some of them several times over several years. These interviews usually lasted about an hour, although some were as short as 15 minutes and the longest was more than 3 hours. All in all, I conducted 130 interviews, most of which were audio recorded and transcribed prior to analysis. (When the person I was talking to preferred I not audio record, which happened a few times, I would take notes during the conversation instead.) Over the following years, I returned several times to Brookfield and Park City. I checked in with the youth I had known as teenagers and interviewed several of them, and sometimes their family members as well, about their transition into adulthood. The initial research was reviewed and approved by the Social and Behavioral Sciences Institutional Review Board at the University of Chicago; the follow-up fieldwork was reviewed and approved by the institutional review board at Duquesne University.

Chapter Summaries

The book begins with my arrival in Brookfield; like many ethnographic arrival stories, it starts with the adoption of awkward new roles at the start of an arduous and potentially transformative quest. The Unity Center, a community organization for youth on the spectrum, was offering a summer camp for these youth in collaboration with the Journeyfolk, a community of live-action role-playing gamers; I came on board as ethnographer, counselor, and fellow sword-wielding adventurer. Chapter 1, "The Summer of Adventure," explores the affinities between the cognitive characteristics associated with autism spectrum conditions and the cultural practices of the Journeyfolk, showing how neurodevelopmental differences take on form, meaning, and valence through shared social practices.

With the end of summer comes the beginning of the school year—and for students on the autism spectrum, a new set of challenges. Chapter 2, "Searching for a Place," follows the fraught journeys of students with Asperger's and related conditions within the bureaucracy of special education, a system that simultaneously individualizes and aggregates them. Through this process, kids learn to identify with the cognitive classifications that determine their tenuous place in the world. Chapter 3, "Innocent Machines," explores what these kids learn about themselves, by examining how the meanings of autism spectrum conditions are negotiated and strategically deployed within two Asperger-specific school programs in Brookfield. Contrasting the appealingly technoscientific Asperger's students with the messy interpersonal entanglements, troubled backgrounds, and moral culpability of students with psychiatric, emotional, and/or behavioral disturbances often worked to preserve a separate space for the Asperger's students and to garner them scarce educational resources. However, this conception of the Asperger's students as "innocent machines" could not effectively conceptualize the moral agency of their robustly social lives.

The distinction between psychiatric "brainhoods" characterized by fluidity and sociomoral entanglement, and developmental disabilities, characterized in contrast as fixed and impervious to social influence, has resonances that transcend the specific politics of the Brookfield school district. Chapter 4, "Hardwired," shifts to the nearby Park City, placing these findings in the broader context of a distinction between the "neurochemical self" as outlined by sociologist Nikolas Rose (2003, 2007) and a "neurostructural self" articulated by individuals affected by autism spectrum conditions. Drawing on observations of a support group run by and for people who identify as having Asperger's syndrome or related autism spectrum conditions, as well as interviews with participants, this chapter describes how conceptualizations of the "neurostructural self" as physiologically fixed can serve as a form of resistance to the imperatives of "fluid modernity" for constant self-optimization, adaptability, and flexibility—demands that are particularly taxing for the types of people who wind up with autism spectrum diagnoses.

The recent move toward conceptualizing neurodevelopment as plastic, however, undermines this distinction, opening new areas of the self-in-the-world to medical intervention. Chapter 5, "The Pathogen and the Package," introduces the contentious topic of physiological prevention of autism, analyzing interviews with Park City autism scientists and national research conference presentations to unpack the multiplicitous ways in which autism as a target of intervention is defined within various medical and scientific practices. Two traditions in contemporary biomedicine—one focused on detecting and eliminating discrete disease entities and the other seeking to map and modulate comprehensive neurogenetic systems—produce different but overlapping "autisms": a "pathogen-like" autism that is separable, exclusively negative, and damaging to the self, on one hand, and a "whole package" autism that is an inseparable and constitutive element of personhood, with both positive and negative aspects, on the other. Through the process mentioned earlier, which I call "divided medicalization," the former comes to stand in for the latter, allowing for the occlusion and potentially the suppression of autism's multivalent, aesthetic, and identitarian dimensions. Chapter 6, "The Division of a Syndrome," demonstrates the process of divided medicalization in action through an ethnographic case study of the formation and dissolution of an Asperger's syndrome clinic located within a university medical center in Park City. Social, aesthetic, and identitarian elements of the condition were at first invited into but then gradually banished from the clinic, leaving behind an incomplete and impoverished representation of Asperger's as a disorder to be eliminated from individuals. Chapter 7, "The Dilemma of Cure," returns to Brookfield to discuss how youth on the spectrum and their families answer the question, *If you could go back in time and get rid of the autism that affects you, would you do it?* Their answers demonstrate how the intractable ethical conflicts around prevention and cure arise out of a particular conception of both autism and personhood as located within bounded individual bodies.

The remaining two chapters of the book provide alternatives: practices that transcend this model to conceptualize and treat social disorder as a phenomenon that occurs in the spaces between us. Chapter 8, "The Sword in the Soul," explores how Brookfield youth diagnosed with autism spectrum conditions draw on folk mythologies of permeable selves to conceptualize their condition. Autism, to them, feels both intimate and alien, brings both cherished strengths and terrifying vulnerability, and constitutes their sense of self while also profoundly disrupting it. They struggle to formulate and express these coexistences through the medicalized languages of pathogenesis and neurogenetic personhood. By playfully reinventing their autobiographies through an alternative shared mythology, however, they generate new ways of coming to terms with the complexities of their condition. The Conclusion, "Bowling Together," ends the book with some recommendations, suggesting that interventions on the social disorder associated with neurodevelopmental difference should attend not only to individual bodies but also to the repair of local connections and the rebuilding of social capital.

About the Writing of This Book

In the process of writing this book, I've made a number of stylistic and representational decisions, each of which has benefits and drawbacks. For example, there are a number of moments in this book where events are depicted in the present tense: *Fred considers his stepson to be . . .* Yet this book is a series of snapshots taken over a number of years in the past—and these are years in the lives of young people, and young people change so very quickly. In my mind, my friend Sylvester, a major character in this book, is still a quicksilver preteen; in reality, he is now an adult, and his feelings and attitudes, as well as those of his family, have likely changed in many ways since our time sword fighting in his backyard garden. As for me, when I began this research, I was a graduate student, fiery and uncertain—now, as I finish it, I am a university professor myself, supervising graduate students on their own research projects while striving for the stability of tenure. In writing this book, I have taken real people—myself included—and made them into book characters, figures who are there to represent and convey particular elements of a story, and, in doing, so have frozen some of the dynamism of their actual lives. I have written in this way to preserve a sense of vividness and immediacy, inviting readers who feel today as the characters in this book have in the past to recognize a little of themselves. But as far as the actual people upon whom this book is based are concerned, know that this use of present tense is a literary convention, a piece of artistic license on my part; time has passed, and they may see things very differently now.

Questions of language in autism are complicated. Some people on the autism spectrum prefer to be referred to using person-first language (Carla is a *person with autism*), while others prefer identity-first language (Carla is *autistic*). I discuss these issues in greater detail later in the book. While I myself incline toward identity-first language, as it is more evocative of autism as I have come to understand it, I use both styles here to represent this diversity of views, following the preference of the person to whom I refer when I know what that is. On the topic of language choices: throughout the book, I use the singular *they* as a gender-neutral pronoun rather than using a phrase such as "he or she." I do so because the range of people to which these pronouns refer includes those, such as gender-nonbinary and genderfluid people, who may not identify either as "he" or as "she."

I have changed the names of all participants, locations, and programs, sometimes changing a few details that might otherwise be identifying. In doing so, I have prioritized concealing the identities of people who shared their lives with me over taking the opportunity to credit by name much of the creative work that has made possible both this book and the communities it depicts. This has been, at moments, a tough choice. My initial reason for saying I would change all identifiers, even of people and programs that might prefer to be named, was because these programs and communities are close together both geographically and socially; naming one would give clues to the identity of all others, which might then lead to individual participants becoming more identifiable. To the extent I can, I have tried to support the work of these programs and people in other ways in other areas of my life and work.

During the same time that I have been gathering, analyzing, and writing up these data, I was also training to become a licensed clinical psychologist. My clinical training has brought me into a number of settings focused on the needs of people on the autism spectrum and their families: several hospitals, a private practice, a special needs summer camp. My experience in these settings has informed my approach to this book, as well as its analysis and conclusions. I was not formally gathering data in any of these settings: I didn't conduct interviews or take field notes, and none of my specific experiences in my clinical practice are shared in this book. But I learned a great deal about both autism spectrum conditions and the experiences of people affected by autism spectrum conditions across a variety of different settings, some of which differ significantly from the contexts where I conducted my research. My training taught me a lot about the kinds of interventions that are currently prevalent within more mainstream educational and treatment settings than those at the center of my research. It also gave me some perspective on the kind of situations that might be specific to Brookfield and Park City versus the kind of situations that seemed to be shared by patients and families in the Midwest and Pacific Northwest where I did my clinical training.

This perspective has been helpful since the research that produced this book does not constitute anything like a representative sample of people on the autism spectrum. While this book focuses on the experience of those who might be described as having "Asperger's syndrome" or "high-functioning autism," it is not a representative sample of these groups either. Both these categories are "moving targets," in Hacking's (2007) sense—their composition and contents are constantly shifting, often in response to social scientific attempts to construct and then intervene upon them. Their boundaries are contested (High-functioning in what way? Under what circumstances? According to whom?), and even their official definitions are in ongoing flux. For all these reasons, developing epidemiological data on the demographic distribution of these conditions has been difficult (Fombonne, 2005; Fombonne & Tidmarsh, 2003).

A few absences, however, are particularly worth recognizing. Of the 50 people I interviewed who identified as being on the autism spectrum, 38 were, to the best of my knowledge, male. This was in keeping with research at the time which found much higher rates of Asperger's syndrome among boys and men than among girls and women (Whiteley, Todd, Carr, & Shattock, 2010; Wilkinson, 2008); since then, however, there has been a growing awareness that women who might benefit from an autism spectrum diagnosis often go undiagnosed, managing to pass or "camouflage" their differences and the challenges they cause (Dean, Hartwood, & Kasari, 2017; Duvekot et al., 2017; Lai et al., 2017). Furthermore, I say "to the best of my knowledge" because I didn't have as clear a sense then as I do now that some of the folks I talked to may not have identified as the gender that they appeared as to me or as the gender corresponding to the pronoun that their parents or teachers used to refer to them. Of the people who participated in this research, only two explicitly identified themselves to me as transgender or nonbinary, possibly because the rest of them didn't experience or define themselves in that way and possibly also because I didn't ask them about it. However, the past years have brought a growing awareness of people on the spectrum who identify as gender-nonconforming in some way (Glidden et al., 2016; van Schalkwyk, Klingensmith, & Volkmar, 2018). Were I doing this research today, more of them would likely show up in the book that came out of it.

For what it's worth, I myself do not identify as a person on the autism spectrum, and I've never been identified as such, although I've also never quite managed to find myself in the word *neurotypical*. Perhaps it goes without saying, but perhaps it is also worth saying, that this is a different book than would be written by someone on the autism spectrum. (I wouldn't venture to speculate about how it would be different without knowing a great deal more about that hypothetical author.) Much of the content of this book and its conclusions are grounded in the insights and conceptual work being done, in talk and practice, by people on the autism spectrum. However, responsibility for the analysis and final conclusions rests with me. Increasing numbers of scholars on the autism spectrum are sharing their own analysis of these and other issues across a variety of venues, and I encourage readers to seek these out according to their own questions and interests (a few of my personal favorites are cited throughout this book, but there are many, many more).

As far as this book goes, I try to illustrate that autism is not only a thing that inheres within labeled individuals but also a thing that happens relationally between people (including those not so labeled). I am writing this book as a person for whom the phenomenon called autism has resonated across a number of arenas: as an open question among friends and lovers about their relationship to normative sociality, interest, and desire; as an energy driving artistic and political projects both constructive and destructive; as a constitutive aspect of my professional life; and as a catalyst for ethical questions, some of which have been profoundly difficult and some of which have been painfully clear. In this sense, I suppose you could say that although I am not an *autistic person*,

I am a *person with autism*, as autism has been with me for lo these many years. The fact that this has been a choice of mine, a matter of affinity, is a definitional aspect of my way of *being with autism*, one that has shaped this book's focus on matters of affinity, attraction, affiliation, and choice. Through these mechanisms, people who are affected by autism in many different ways come together and create cultural spaces; those spaces provide the context for this book and the stories it tells.

1

The Summer of Adventure

I Could Write You a Kind of Low-Impact Character If You Wanted

When Elise invited me to come to Staff Week, I had a few preconceived notions about what awaited me there.[1] Trainings. Suit jackets. Conference rooms. Artsy adults in chunky jewelry. PowerPoint presentations about best practices for autism whose slides I could potentially analyze in hopes of extracting their underlying logics. Maybe some team-building exercises; maybe some kind of a ropes course.

I had arranged to start the research for my PhD dissertation by spending 6 months conducting ethnographic participant observation at the Unity Center, a community center serving youth with Asperger's syndrome and related autism spectrum conditions. Elise, one of the two co-directors, suggested that I come a few months early to help at the summer camp they were running that summer for youth on the spectrum, in collaboration with a local group called the Journeyfolk. She invited me to start by attending their Staff Week to learn a bit more about what the group did. So I made sure to pack a bunch of suit jackets near the top of the suitcases filling my aging Volkswagen and drove it to the East Coast from Chicago, stopping only to get the steering system repaired when it gave out on the way. *I'm doing fieldwork,* I wrote eagerly in my notebook as I sat in the car repair shop waiting room, somewhere deep in Pennsylvania. *I'm really, really, doing it. Fieldwork.*

"Turn off the main road when you see signs for the Coller Center," Elise had told me. "Drive through the woods until you see people. Then ask for Michael." Down the twisty road I drove, through the trees, an alarmingly long way, until I came to a clearing. A few teenagers were hanging around, looking like they belonged there: a long-legged girl with long red hair, a gangly kid folded up by a picnic table, a young man with hair in locs and a streak of shimmering green traced across the bridge of his pierced nose. They stared with moderate interest. I asked for Michael, and they pointed down the road, giving slow, sardonic claps as I awkwardly maneuvered the car around to the right direction.

Michael, a fellow who seemed to be in his mid-20s, was giving instructions to a bunch of younger folks unloading big boxes of food and trying to find places to put them (there was some kind of problem with the refrigerator). He greeted me warmly and helped me get settled. I was welcome to use his tent, he offered, since he wasn't going to be using it, or I could find a bed in one of the cabins. Not having packed for camping, I opted for the latter and found myself sharing a room with two teenage girls who were very nice and very eager to make me feel welcome. "I used to be, like, a video game person," one of the girls said to me. She meant that her interest in video games had once shielded her from a fuller engagement with social life. "I used to be a pushover." She wanted me to understand what this community had done for her. "You don't know how brave you can be until you've had the chance to do something brave."

The Journeyfolk, among whom I had found myself, are a close-knit collective of young people dedicated to transforming themselves and building community through the art of live-action role-playing games. These games combine elements of collaborative storytelling, improvisational theater, and tabletop games of the Dungeons and Dragons sort. Their busiest time is the summer, when they run a series of "Summer of Adventure" camps—one of which, this year, was the "Aspie Camp" developed in collaboration with the Unity Center. But there are many camps, most of which aren't focused around a particular neurodevelopmental type: an Intro Camp for new players, an Advanced Camp for those more experienced, a Journeykids camp for littler kids. Once you turn 16, you can apply to be an SIT, or Staffer-In-Training. Staff Week, I discovered, is when the SITs get together with the older counselors to learn the ropes, and to run a little wild before stepping into their new positions as role models for younger kids.

On the third day of Staff Week, we had a Game. Energy was crackling in the air as the Journeyfolk bounced from building to building, talking fast, borrowing each other's jewelry and donning elaborate costumes, and setting up props and scenery in a series of locations all over the

Coller Center grounds. All the staff—the SITs and the counselors—had been assigned to role-play particular characters, whose intersecting histories, conflicts, goals, and motivations would create the drama that would unfold. We had witnessed a teaser for the game, a brief, starkly lit scene during which a captured gangster had been tortured, interrogated, and shot (Staff Week games could get pretty intense). The story writer for that week's Game had created a scenario and a "flow" of events to take place throughout the night, giving certain players enough information that they could set those events in motion and, in some cases, giving them the explicit responsibility for doing so. Unsure what to do with myself, I found the story writer and asked her where would be a good place to sit and watch the game that night.

She gave me a look. It was a look I had been getting a lot over the past few days. It wasn't a mean look; it was just a bit alarmed and confused. It told me I had just said something that made absolutely no sense.

"Well," she replied, "I could write you a kind of low-impact character if you wanted."

So I dug out a wrinkled suit jacket from where it had fallen to the bottom of my bag and spent the night as a member of the Trinidad Mafia. I spent a lot of time sitting around with my fellow Mafiosi as we made despicable plans, and attempting an accent that I eventually jettisoned. The whole thing was completely overwhelming. My field notes from the following day about the game summarized it merely as "a lot of gunfire and torture and lost love" and "I feel dazed."

Fortunately, the next day—as was protocol among the Journey-folk—we all sat around and told the stories we had lived the night before. I had experienced the game from the vantage point of a Mafiosa; the other groups in the game saw different stories unfold. There was no single vantage point from which to observe the game; more stories were always happening than any one person could see or tell. Through this communal storytelling, a bit more of a collective sense of the night's events gradually emerged—something like what cultural psychologist Rick Shweder (2003) would call a "view from manywheres." Deceptions were revealed; heartbreaks were processed. Story is the stuff that life among the Journeyfolk is made of.

I was glad I had a costume easily at hand; other than that, I was utterly unprepared for the situation I had found my way into. I had come to the Journeyfolk camp as the first piece of a 2-year comparative ethnographic study on programs for youth with Asperger's syndrome. I had not initially planned on casting spells, evading assassins, or spending the evening as a different person than I had woken up as that morning. Furthermore, I had come to the Journeyfolk camp carrying a lot of implicit expectations, expectations carried with me from my clinical training, about what a therapeutic intervention involving Asperger's syndrome would look like: controlled environments, clear role differentiations between patients and therapists, the ability to go home at the end of the day. That being said, I had known that I was in for something a little different when I came to the Unity Center. The group of educators who had formed the Unity Center had done so, in part, because they weren't satisfied with existing approaches to autism. They wanted to change the way we think about what autism is, and the way we respond to it.

Several years earlier, the mother of a boy diagnosed with Asperger's syndrome, Mariel Mattheson, had become intrigued by the possibilities of autistic culture. A few years later, she herself would be diagnosed with Asperger's as well. Inspired by the nascent neurodiversity movement, and its roots within autistic self-advocacy, she wondered how her son's struggles in school might change if he were among other autistic students in an environment that treated his condition not as a disorder but as a valued difference. In collaboration with the local school district, she opened a classroom along these principles, which I will call ASPIRE.

Both the original name of the program and the pseudonym I have chosen play on the word *Asperger's*. However, the Asperger's diagnosis here was less of a formal criterion for acceptance into the program and more of a prototype for its spirit: Participants in the program had a wide range of autism spectrum diagnoses, from "high-functioning autism" to PDD-NOS. The word *Asperger's* was used to highlight the extent to which these students had numerous intact or even extraordinary abilities to go along with the vulnerabilities that were disabling to them. The students were those on the expanding edges of the autism spectrum: significantly challenged by their social difficulties and tendency toward routine, repetition, and rigidity while lacking the significant cognitive and language impairments long associated with autism. ASPIRE approached autism spectrum disorders as bringing strengths to be celebrated and challenges to be managed, explicitly rejecting the idea that they are diseases to be cured. Its curriculum was designed not only to teach traditional academic skills but also to build self-esteem, self-advocacy, and a sense of culture and community among young people on the autism spectrum.

ASPIRE was therefore a program on the leading edge of many of the issues I hoped to explore in my own research, and I contacted Mariel to see if I could conduct research there. She was supportive of the project and welcomed my interest. However, she told me, after the ASPIRE program had been in operation for 2 years the school district had opted not to continue it. Unwilling to give up on the community that had formed around the school and its principles, Mariel and her collaborator, Elise, had then opened a community center, the Unity Center, and were in the process of converting it to a small private school. I arranged with them to spend 6 months conducting participant observation once the school opened, which I would then contrast with 6 months at a more standard clinic housed within a nearby medical school, with the aim of comparing "cultural" and "medical" models of autism as they played out in practice.[2] I arrived 2 months early to help out with their summer camp.

The physical education teacher at ASPIRE, Mark, had been one of the original founders of the Journeyfolk Collective. After ASPIRE closed, Mark and the Journeyfolk started offering programming at the Unity Center on weekends. Both at ASPIRE and at the regular Journeyfolk camps, Mark had observed that campers with Asperger's often seemed to respond to the game in a special way. "The kids with Asperger's tend to really get—as we called it—*into character*," Mark told me. "They really could embody a character. Because I think they really could imagine, identify—and *had* identified, through their reading or fascination with fantasy literature or video games. And they could understand how to be that character. More than, sometimes, kids who would be, you know—quote-unquote *normal*." But many of these youth also became overwhelmed by the immersive social life of the sleepaway camps and needed more support than the staff there could provide. So the Journeyfolk designed a small day camp with a high staff-to-camper ratio targeted particularly toward "Aspie" campers, in collaboration with the Unity Center; this year was its second year.

At first glance, it seems remarkable that the role-playing games designed by Mark and the Journeyfolk would be so appealing for youth on the autism spectrum. After all, these games required them to do many of the things that are said to be most difficult for people on the autism spectrum: taking another person's perspective, stepping (literally!) into someone else's shoes and acting as that character would in a particular situation, using nonverbal communication to show other players how their character feels and to create lively interactions, collaborating with others in an elaborate shared mental representation. The game thus posed distinct challenges for those on the autism spectrum; however, it also provided a distinctive array of inviting sociocultural resources to support them. Understanding why the Aspie campers so loved the Game, therefore, requires that we understand not only their individual cognitive vulnerabilities but also how they make use of the rich array of affordances offered them by their cultural worlds.

You Can Go Hunting With a Knife and Fork

A significant body of research in psychology has attempted to identify the cognitive differences underlying the profile of behavioral and experiential characteristics that co-occur in autism. Researchers increasingly acknowledge that no one theory will explain all aspects of autism and that not all people with an autism spectrum diagnosis will fit any one description (Brunsdon & Happé, 2014; Vanegas & Davidson, 2015). However, several theories have received significant empirical support and attention. Most prominent have been those related to limitations in theory of mind (the ability to conceptualize and reason about other people's internal states; e.g., Baron-Cohen, 1995; Kana, Libero, Hu, Deshpande, & Colburn, 2012), executive function (the ability to organize and manage one's cognitive processes in a flexible way; e.g., Craig et al., 2016; Ozonoff, Pennington, & Rogers, 1991; Ozonoff, Strayer, McMahon, & Filloux, 1994; Pennington & Ozonoff, 1996), and bias toward local over global coherence (in other words, a tendency to focus on details, and calculate precise relationships between those details rather than synthesizing them intuitively into a big-picture gestalt; e.g., Happé & Frith, 2006).

The most well-known theory of autism proposes that people diagnosed with autism are experiencing a deficit in *theory of mind*, or what Baron-Cohen (1995) has called "mindblindness." Numerous studies have documented that people with this cognitive profile have difficulty correctly attributing mental states (beliefs, desires, intentions, etc.) to others, especially when those mental states are different from their own (see Frith, 2012, for a review). Consequently, the behavior and reactions of others often appear to be capricious, incomprehensible, and generally unpredictable. Drawing on this theory, Baron-Cohen, Richler, Bisarya, Gurunathan, and Wheelwright (2003) have suggested that a preference for systematizing (analyzing variables in a system to discern their underlying rules) over empathizing (intuitively inferring the internal states of others) may be fundamental to the autistic cognitive style, arguing that some of the social struggles experienced by people on the autism spectrum result from an oft-thwarted search to find the systems that reliably predict human behavior.

Another well-known theory involves *executive function* (Ozonoff et al., 1991, 1994; Pennington & Ozonoff, 1996; Robinson, Goddard, Dritschel, Wisley, & Howlin, 2009). Executive function is commonly compared to the conductor of an orchestra; it is the brain function that coordinates other brain functions so that they work together smoothly and efficiently toward a goal. Individuals on the autism spectrum often show difficulty planning and carrying out tasks in the absence of external structure, difficulty in flexibly shifting approaches when task demands change, and a vulnerability to extreme fluctuations in mood, all signs of executive dysfunction. Contributing to their overall difficulty organizing their experience, individuals on the autism spectrum often struggle to process and integrate sensory input—sounds, smells, tastes, the brightness of light, and the babble of voices in a crowd (Baranek, David, Poe, Stone, & Watson, 2006; Baranek, 2002; Dunn, Saiter, & Rinner, 2002). This overwhelmed state can lead to the "meltdowns" often observed in individuals on the autism spectrum: a loss of behavioral control, characterized by aggression, manifestations of intense distress, and/or profound, frozen withdrawal (Myles, 2003; Myles & Southwick, 1999).

Individuals on the autism spectrum are also often said to display what has alternately been called *weak central coherence* or a preference for *local over global coherence* (Happé & Frith, 2006). In other words, when taking in a scene, individuals with this perceptual style tend to focus on individual details and local, clearly observable relationships between those details, rather than displaying the more typical perceptual style of integrating details into a fuzzier "big picture" and making inferences about higher order meaning ("central" or "global coherence"). In some cases, a locally coherent processing style can increase the accuracy of perception. For example, individuals on the autism spectrum have been shown to perform better than typically developing individuals on tasks requiring them to pick figures out of a distracting context (de Jonge, Kemner, & van Engeland, 2006; Joliffe & Baron-Cohen, 1997). Sometimes, however, attention to local relationships can mean missing the proverbial forest for the trees. In another study, for example, subjects with a pronounced local-coherent style were more likely than those with a more typical, global-coherent style to complete sentence stems in a way that did not make sense in their broader context, for example, completing the stem "You can go hunting with a knife and . . ." with "fork" rather than with something like "kill a wild beast" (Booth & Happé, 2010). Focusing on details rather than on integrating those details into a big picture can produce what researcher Uta Frith (1989, p. 98) memorably described as "an incoherent world of fragmented experience." As long as it is the local relationship between individual items that constitutes the nature of the whole, rather than a less precise and more robust conceptualization of its overall gestalt, small changes in the relationship between items destabilize the continuity and basic nature of the entire system. Moving a piece of furniture in a room, changing the order of tasks on a schedule, taking different turns on the drive home—these alternations that might seem insignificant to those with a more globally coherent style can produce a sense of deep ontological uncertainty, an existential sort of distress in those who are processing locally. This vulnerability motivates an attentive care for local relationships, making a priority of their intact preservation.

The autistic cognitive style, and particularly the challenges that come with it, have traditionally been depicted as a series of individual deficits in executive function, theory of mind, and central coherence: as inabilities to organize, to intuit, and to infer, without explicit guidance. Some of the research on cognition in autism has been less deficit-focused, depicting these cognitive differences as a difference in style rather than a lack. For example, Laurent Mottron and his research team (Mottron, Dawson, Soulieres, Hubert, & Burack, 2006), which includes scientists on the autism spectrum, have suggested that autistic cognition is characterized by a pattern of enhancements in perceptual processing (see also Baron-

Cohen, 2000; Happé & Frith, 2006). Overall, however, the research on cognition in autism has sought to locate the origins of what manifests as autism exclusively within the individual minds of those diagnosed.

To understand what was going on at the Journeyfolk camp, however—as well as the questions that are posed by this book more broadly—we need to engage instead with the ways that human cognition is inextricable from culture, and the possibility that the kind of cognitive processes that get labeled "autistic," rather than being exceptions to this rule, are instead exemplars of it. All these different theories, in their own ways, describe an inconstant and unpredictable phenomenological world, threatened perpetually by chaos, disorganization, and the breakdown of meaning—an internal experience deeply reliant on external structure to fend off these threats. What if we were thus to consider theory of mind, executive function, and the creation of coherence not as individualized processes but as collaborative engagements with the stuff of culture? Anthropologist Clifford Geertz (2000) describes culture as a web of interconnected symbols, "a set of control mechanisms—plans, recipes, rules, instructions (what computer engineers call 'programs')—for the governing of behavior" without which "man's behavior would be virtually ungovernable, a mere chaos of pointless acts and exploding emotions, his experience virtually shapeless" (p. 44). Human beings, he suggests in his essay "The Impact of the Concept of Culture on the Concept of Man," are "the animal most desperately dependent on such extragenetic, outside-the-skin control mechanisms, such cultural programs, for ordering their behavior. . . . We are, in sum, incomplete or unfinished animals who complete or finish ourselves through culture" (p. 49).

People who exhibit the cognitive style described earlier make particularly active use of existing cultural material to organize and order their experience, make predictions and inferences, and plan and govern behavior. They are, to use Geertz's formulation, particularly dependent on culture to complete them. These extrasomatic arrangements, these existing sets of relationships between particular items, are taken in whole cloth and used to provide order, stability, and comfort to an unpredictable phenomenological world. The relationship with formal structure among many people who receive autism spectrum diagnoses is aesthetic, intimate, desperate, protective, and profound. The threat of fragmentation—fragmentation of the self, of the world, and of the tenuous connections between—lurks always in the shifting movements of time, space, and relationships. Continuity in these domains is an accomplishment, one which must be regularly renewed and actively maintained. These processes are thus intimately co-constituted by the affordances of surrounding meaning-worlds.

I Want to Tell You a Story

Different cultural resources and practices offer different kinds of support for this process. Given its importance, this is a factor significantly understudied in autism, where much of the most influential research has been carried out within laboratories and other research settings that have been designed to control and minimize external sources of variance. Such a process is not likely to foreground the ways in which cognitive processes are shaped by rich and varied human environments. However, other research projects (many of which are outside the disciplines of psychology and psychiatry) have taken up this question directly. In their Ethnography of Autism Project, linguistic anthropologist Elinor Ochs and her research team (Ochs, Kremer-Sadlik, Sirota, & Solomon, 2004) conducted several years of in-depth ethnographic observation of children with high-functioning autism in their daily lives: video recording and micro-analyzing their interactions with family members during dinnertimes and other shared moments, looking for conditions of interactional success as well as failure. They found that the children were most successful in situations organized around a "stable symbolic and social order, of rules, schemata, and structural features" (p. 172). The children struggled, however, with the kinds of social practices that required "intuitively formulating strategies for interpreting and participating in emergent yet conventional social situations" (p. 148). Family members were able to help scaffold ongoing conversations that might otherwise disintegrate into chaos; certain social forms (those somewhat fixed and stable in their form, such as a question–answer pair or a shared and explicit moral rule) offered support as well. The result is an orientation toward cultural practices that provide such explicit conventions, remaining stable and predictable while providing an array of interlinked contextual cues about their meanings and expectations. For example, Solomon (2004, p. 260) found that, compared to typically developing kids as well as to their other family members, children on the spectrum were more likely to tell "prepackaged" fictional narratives taken from movies or television, rather than relate events from their own life. They were often able to launch fictional narratives successfully, partly because of the conventionalized language often used to begin such stories (e.g., "I want to tell you a story about [topic]"), although they struggled to maintain a collaborative "co-telling" with a listener across multiple conversational turns. Solomon suggests that the preorganization of events already "extracted from the experiential flow" and placed into "stable temporal and causal trajectories" (p. 260) relieves children of some of the organizational burden of creating coherence. Such research, she wrote in a later review in *Annual Reviews in Anthropology*, "suggests that sociality, and by extension executive function, in autism is less a property of the individual and more a property of social interaction" (Solomon, 2010, p. 251). Successful social coordination depends on the generosity of particular environments and particular interlocutors.

As an assemblage of practices and cultural materials, live-action role-playing games provide an array of resources that are a good fit for these needs (see Fein, 2015). Role-playing games offload the pressure to extract and organize salient social information by placing numerous components of social life into a shared, stable, and explicit narrative framework. In the preparation phase for the game, which at the Aspie Camp took up the first 3 days of each week, players are presented with a "story intro" that describes the world where the story takes place and delineates some of its salient social dynamics. The expectation is that information shared in this way will be acted on, and acted out, within the game's interactions. Consequently, selected elements of social interaction are extracted, highlighted, and prioritized in advance, lessening the demand to make these distinctions in the moment. Furthermore, characters in the game have quantified amounts of certain qualities (such as strength, wisdom, dexterity, and charisma), and these traits have causal force in character interactions: If a character with high charisma asks your character to do something, respect for the game system entails that your character do it. In addition to the explicit game rules, character behavior and interaction in-game are also shaped by a widely known set of genre conventions drawn from fantasy literature and swords-and-sorcery games. Adherence to these conventions organized interactions in-game, by imposing an external, familiar, shared constraint on conversational possibilities while providing flexible scripts. Social interactions in-game are therefore structured by a top-down, explicitly articulated, systematic, and shared set of behavioral norms and obligations—the very kind of system that is most productive of interactive success among individuals on the spectrum.

This structure facilitated the "sustained co-telling" of narratives that Solomon (2004) identified as most difficult for youth on the spectrum. I often marveled at the long back-and-forth conversations, so different from our fragmented out-of-game interactions, that I had with the Aspie campers when we were in character. The congruence between the organization of role-playing games and the needs of people with Asperger's provided both motivation to participate in these games and support for successful social coordination within them. The campers were therefore able to have experiences that were not as common in the chaos and confusion of their everyday lives: They could be valued contributors, both to their team of fellow heroic adventurers and to the greater project of creating the story as a whole.

This Weird Urge to Stand Up and Say: These Are My People

The extent to which autism spectrum conditions were appreciated by the Journeyfolk highlights the way neurodevelopmental difference manifests and takes on its valence in particular contexts, even as it is often described as a feature of particular minds. The camp provided an opportunity to step away from mainstream culture and into an environment where different social and cognitive demands reconfigured profiles of ability and disability. As numerous scholars of disability (e.g., Ingstad & Whyte, 1995; Varenne & McDermott, 1995; see also the work of ethnomusicologist Michael Bakan, 2014, 2018) have argued, cultures themselves can be disabling—or enabling—for particular members, and the nature of a disability depends very much on the particular demands and opportunities of the given environment. The Journeyfolk were a subculture with their own distinct set of norms, of which they were very proud. (Upon being told that a camper had in the past been hospitalized due to losing the ability to discriminate between fantasy and reality, one of the counselors laughed, "Oh, we don't mind *that!*"). Among the Journeyfolk, social life is organized around the Game, and the capacities that lead to a good game are highly prized. In the alternative cultural setting of the Journeyfolk, characteristics common to many people with Asperger's syndrome—their consciously learned social behaviors, their ability to put aside informal social norms, their appreciation for genre structure and formality, their ability to imagine themselves as figures out of a written text—were not seen as impairments or symptoms but, rather, were valued and appreciated for their unique contributions to gameplay.

"That's what made me fall in love with the Aspie [program]," Evie pointed out in one of the first team meetings of the Aspie Camp staff. "The intensity of interest. The *noooooblenenss* of the heroes." Evie was in her mid-20s, with a pair of pointy pigtails and a radiant grin. Involved with the Journeyfolk since her early teens, she now held a leadership position in the organization and was working with Mark to lead the Aspie Camp. She had a way of zigzagging through the world like a bolt of lightning, never staying too long in any one spot. But Evie was no stranger to deep commitments—much of her life was devoted to the world and work of the Journeyfolk, even as she barely made enough money doing it to keep herself fed and tenuously housed. Also, she knew every word of the film *Casablanca* by heart. The staff of the Aspie Camp seemed generally to share that combination of deep, near-obsessive interests and easygoing disregard for mainstream social expectations.

At the start of the camp, our staff consisted of Howard and Evie, and veteran Journeyfolk counselors Patrick, Clyde, Jenna, and William. (A few folks switched in and out as the summer went on.) We were also joined by Imogen, a longtime Journeyfolk camper diagnosed with Asperger's; witnessing her deep immersion into character had been one of Mark's early inspirations for creating Asperger-specific programming. Mark had invited her to help with the camp and she graduated to being a full staff member in its second half. I participated in multiple capacities: as counselor, ethnographer, role-player, and occasional clinical consultant.

The staff of the Unity Center were also around. Elise often joined us for meetings. Annie was a volunteer at Unity who took care of a lot of what needed to get done around the center on a day-to-day basis. Her son, Sylvester, was diagnosed with high-functioning autism; he loved the Journeyfolk games and the Unity Center community, and she planned to enroll him in the center's school when it opened in the fall. Eleven years old, with a mop of brown hair and green eyes that tilted like a cat's, he was a little sprite that danced from playful to furious in the span of a heartbeat. The previous year, he'd been suspended from school for the first time—he had been so out of control that it had taken three full-sized adults to restrain him. "Sometimes Sylvester doesn't even know when he's upset about something," Elise explained ruefully to Mark and me. Then she laughed. "Which is why he gets so upset about things!"

While Imogen was the only staff member explicitly identified as being on the autism spectrum, the staff, on the whole, did not identify as being particularly neurotypical. "Patrick and Clyde are so talented they're almost Asperger's themselves," Mark once observed admiringly. Encountering the notion of autism as a spectrum, rather than an all-or-nothing category that you are in or you are out of, something you have or you do not, was intriguing to the staff. It changed the way they thought about both the condition and themselves. "I'm glad Elise explained that I can have Asperger's *traits*," Clyde said after our first meeting. Many of the staff members reported feeling a sense of commonality, loyalty, and kinship with the campers, even as they also recognized the way in which the campers were facing challenges more extreme, for the most part, than their own social struggles had been. "They're my *tribe*," Patrick enthused in a group meeting. When I asked him to explain what he meant, he elaborated:

> Because we're interested in some of the same things: video games, role-playing, fantasy, things like that. And I was always identified as being a nerd. If I walk into a room and there's a table with people wearing nice clothing, chilling, drinking beer—I'm gonna go to the little group of guys in the corner playing Magic cards. That's where my core goes to. That's where I feel most comfortable. There is something tribal about it, it's very strange. . . . There's a sense of unfairness to it. That I get to do all the things that they do, play all the games that they play—and I also get to go talk to people, and they don't. Something happened to them where they don't get that luxury, of being able to shut that part of you down and go interact with the rest of the world. So I almost feel in a way this weird urge to defend them, to stand up and say: these are *my people*.

As research on the "broader autism phenotype" has shown (Baron-Cohen, Wheelwright, Skinner, Martin, & Clubely, 2001; Constantino &

Todd, 2003; Wheelwright, Auyeung, Allison, & Baron-Cohen, 2010), the cognitive style associated with autism spectrum conditions—relative strength in systematic thinking and relative weakness in social intuition, a focus on local detail over global gestalt, a tendency to focus on a single topic rather than shifting fluidly between topics, and a vulnerability to extreme mood states—occurs along a spectrum that begins long before the point at which these characteristics cause clinically significant impairment. Dispersed through the general population, these characteristics organize people around particular cultural practices—in this case, the structured sociality, artful juxtapositions, rewards for deep commitment, and archetypal, opposing-forces narrative aesthetic of story games ranging from collectible card games such as Magic: The Gathering all the way up to the enacted stories of the Journeyfolk camp. Many of the characteristics shared by the Aspie campers—hyperfocus on a topic of interest, discomfort with unstructured or implicitly structured sociality, an intense and high-contrast but often private emotional ethos, and a pull toward structured, genre-based cultural materials— were also common in the social community that surrounded the Journeyfolk. While these characteristics might be socially stigmatized in mainstream culture as "geeky," they were not understood by the Journeyfolk counselors as inherently problematic; rather, they were woven into a set of cultural practices and celebrated as sources of pleasure, affiliation, and pride. Consequently, characteristics that might elsewhere be read as symptoms of a disorder were reinterpreted as signs of shared belonging within a community.

The Beast of Judgment, the Dark at the End of Everything

At the start of the camp, we were captivated by our commonalities—the Journeyfolk staff with the Aspie campers, the Aspie campers with each other. By the second week of camp, we were working hard to overcome and make room for our differences. Even the seemingly tireless Patrick was starting to get a little worn out. The first week of camp, we had three campers—the second week, we had nine, all older teens, many already familiar with the Journeyfolk games and coming in with a clear sense of what they wanted out of the experience. "Last week I was giving thirty-three and a third percent of myself to each camper," Patrick said. "And that was fine because there were three. Now, I'm still giving thirty-three and a third percent of myself to each camper, but there are nine."

Also, the nine of them had gotten a collective bug in their bonnet about Pirates Versus Ninjas. In a battle between pirates and ninjas, who would win? The campers could, and did, elaborate on this theme and its variations (What about apples versus oranges? Cats versus elephants?) as extensively as the day is long. Meanwhile, Patrick had painstakingly created a beautiful, elaborate story world for the game, led by a well-balanced structure of gods (two brother–sister pairs) and divine animals (the Pig of Dreams, the Bull of Honor, the Fox of Cunning, the Eagle of Courage, and so on). There was not a whole lot of room for Pirates Versus Ninjas. "Which is such a tired old joke," Patrick griped, "and it's all because pirates and ninjas would never encounter each other, hardee har har." Pause. "And besides, pirates would win. But anyway . . ."

Anyway, the campers all had some strong ideas about what they wanted to bring to the game and were not too keen on modifying those ideas to fit the context Patrick provided. They wanted to play characters hailing from a variety of sources and genres—the Legend of Zelda, Pokémon, their own in-jokes and deeply elaborated fantasy worlds. And they liked creating characters that were superpowerful, unbeatable. Losing *anything*—a sword fight, a gold coin out of a pocket, a valued character attribute—was very, very hard for them to bear. As our storywriter, Patrick had gone from taking a professional's pride in how well he could accommodate them—"Anything they throw at me, I can take!" he had bragged in an early staff meeting—to feeling like his job was to keep telling them no, no, no, and then to deal with the explosiveness of their misery. This was less fun of a challenge.

It's the first day of our 2-day Game, at the end of Week 2. We've all been staying at the country house of one of the campers' parents, in a guest room accessible only by ladder. The game will be run on the land all around it, territory that nobody knows all that well. Everyone is exhausted. Patrick, his face still smeared with gaunt shadows of makeup from last night's game back at the main campground, is running through the plan for this day's game. There are four gods and six animals, posted at stations around the land that all nine campers will rotate through. The Eagle of Courage will be down by the shale pit. The Pig of Dreams will be in the meadow. It's all a little confusing.

"Cunning can be at the crossroads, the little crossroads over there by the garden."

"Which one?"

"There's only one crossroads!"

"The one by the barn?"

"No, not that one."

Mark sighs. "I just don't see how it all hangs together. I can't memorize all this stuff. You can, right?" Patrick nods. "It's not the way my brain works."

Patrick keeps running down the list as I frantically try to take notes. As Lady of Twilight, I'm going to take them on a walk through the dark with their eyes closed, following my voice. When they open their eyes, they'll be facing a mirror. The Fox of Cunning is going to give them riddles to solve. The Lord of the Sky hurls thunderbolts for them to dodge as they jump on a trampoline.

"What happens when they get to the Pig of Dreams?" someone asks.

Patrick grins, a beam of light breaking through the shadows. "The Pig is going to challenge them to the Oldest Game."

The Oldest Game goes like this:

I am the fire that consumes and destroys all before me.

I am the water that quenches the fire, leaving nothing behind but a trace of smoke.

Two players face off. The first player declares that they are some powerful force; it is then the other player's turn to declare that they are something that can defeat it. Then it is the first player's turn to transform again.

I am the drought that parches away the water beneath the hot summer sun.

I am the changing of seasons, the blessed relief brought by time and the falling of rain.

The game is built out of the tension between improvisation and form, requiring both inventiveness and the capacity to work within a particular set of parameters. Each transformation must be described as vividly as possible and be closely related to the previous turn (in other words, don't try to fight a fly with an atom bomb). If you hesitate, you lose.

I don't know if this is actually the Oldest Game. It does bear some resemblance to a very old mythological trope, the Transformation Chase,[3] in which one shape-shifter pursues another as they take various forms.

But the term *Oldest Game* comes from modern mythmaker Neil Gaiman (1989), who put a round of it in one of his Sandman comics. The Sandman, otherwise known as Morpheus or just Dream, is in Hell, battling the demon Choronion to recover his stolen helmet. If he wins, he recovers his lost powers; if he loses, he will be forever the plaything of Hell.

I am a dire-wolf, prey-stalking, lethal prowler, the demon Choronion begins the challenge.

I am a hunter, horse-mounted, wolf-stabbing, Dream replies.

And so they continue, in a battle that ranges from a tiny, lethal bacterium up to the world that nurtures life itself.

I am the Universe, Dream states, *all things encompassing, all life embracing.*

The demon replies: *I am anti-life, the beast of judgment. I am the dark at the end of everything. The end of universes, gods, worlds . . . of everything.* He gives a hiss. *And what will you be then, Dreamlord?*

Dream defeats the demon with one simple phrase:

I am Hope (pp. 16–20).

"A fear of death," writes neuroscientist Matthew Belmonte (2008), "drives us to become narrators, to transform the disconnected chaos of our sensorium into representative mental texts whose distinct scenes contain recognizable characters that act in coherent plots and evince meaningful themes" (p. 166). Referencing the work of Ernest Becker, he suggests that the denial of death "can be more generally construed as an aversion to direct experience of disorder and impermanence—the death of the self being an ultimate, personal manifestation of this universal tendency" (p. 166). Drawing on his experience both as a cognitive scientist studying autism and as the brother of someone significantly affected by it, Belmonte suggests that "in this regard, people with autism can be described as 'human but more so': confronted by the same fundamental problem of organizing perceptual experience into coherent stories that confronts all of us, they must overcome greater fragmentation of perceptual and cognitive experience to solve this problem" (p. 173).

What is produced is a different kind of narrative system: one in which the relationship between local, component parts is primary and the emergent gestalt is vulnerable to disruption in any one of those parts. Belmonte (2008) goes on to say that precisely because the narrative defense against sensory chaos is so impaired in autism, people with autism are unusually sensitive to the problem of constructing this defense, and their solutions to this problem tend to be more deliberate and explicit than the rest of us implement. . . . This meticulous, systematic engineering approach to making sense of the world gives rise to a fundamental difference in the quality of autistic thought and the process by which autistic people establish abstract or global relationships: where others may begin with the concept and work down to the details, people with autism study each local detail in isolation, and work up through interactions to the concept. (p. 170)[4]

Through narrative, we propose the radical possibility of meaning. We do so by placing things into relation with other things—by making use of symbols to hold open simultaneously the possibility of *something* and *something else*, along with the idea that there is some possibility of movement between the two for us as conceptual beings. That bridge, the possibility that this bridge is consistent in some way, and the possibility that it be shared with others all provide some alternative to the existential threats of meaninglessness, isolation, and entropy—the deathly threat that "rumbles continuously under the membrane of life" (May & Yalom, 1989, p. 273).

For those on the autism spectrum, however, it often seems that the threat is closer and that the defense is less internal and more collaborative—and yet also more fraught, because it is in collaboration with other people that the structure is held, but it is also in collaboration with other people that the structure changes. Alterations to a piece of the story pose an existential threat, because this intrusion abruptly compromises the integrity of the whole order of one's experiential world. Under such conditions, the mutually responsive co-creation of a story, that experience which the Journeyfolk offer, is an act of enormous bravery.

The Journeyfolk prided themselves on being improvisers and collaborators; the thrill of not knowing what your fellow players would add to the story was part of the fun. Each time a game is run, with the same basic setup manifesting through different players in a different place, a very different set of things will probably happen. The ex-lovers who are joyously reunited in one go-round might, in the next, both be murdered by assassins before they even meet. The king may not reclaim the throne. At least in the more advanced games, the monsters might win. The ability to embrace such uncertainty is a strength the Journeyfolk cultivate. "Flying by the seat of our pants is *part* of the lesson plan," Mark explained patiently to Elise once when she was trying to get them to articulate the goals and objectives for that day's workshop. This dialectic is what the Journeyfolk community is founded on: the generative tension between shared myths and genre conventions, a shared story structure, and a set of stable elements, on one hand, and then the improvisation, the act of co-creation of a particular story, what these elements produced *this time*, on the other. But for the Aspie campers, allowing someone else to alter pieces of your story was a risk far more vulnerable and terrifying, and the stakes were very high. At the Aspie Camp, in a context where people came together around a shared interest and a form of creative play, autism was no longer characterized by isolation and singularity—what Doug Biklen (2005) refers to as "the myth of the person alone." Instead, the challenges we faced had to do with the pain and terror of relatedness, of letting someone else in.

The Little Kids Are Emo

The third and fourth weeks of the camp were for younger teens—the new campers were 11 to 14 or so, although some of them seemed a lot younger. A few of the first weeks' campers remained with us, advancing to the role of counselors-in-training (CITs). As CITs, they were given new responsibilities, ranging from setting a good example for the younger campers to helping with sets, props, and costumes. The shift from camper to CIT also entailed a shift from playing PCs, or "player characters"—adventurer-protagonists of their own design—to playing SPCs, or "staff player characters"—characters whose main purpose was to facilitate a good game for the campers, often by challenging them as adversaries. They thus went from playing their own heroes to playing other people's monsters.[5] It was a lot of responsibility, and it got handed to them very fast.

The first day was a disaster. The big CITs loomed menacingly over the little campers, who saw them as hairy, scary, and mean. When the CITs ran at them waving swords, they were terrified. "I feel *very unhappy!*" Danny, one of the new campers, wept in our closing circle. (He'd clearly spent a lot of time learning to talk about his feelings). We asked the CITs to tone down their monsters, to make them less aggressive and frightening. "What, are we supposed to be, like, *happy monsters*?" they guffawed and then broke into derisive singing. "We're the monsters, the happy happy monsters . . ."

But as nervous as the teens made the little kids, the little kids freaked the teens out way worse. While the older campers were indeed able, as we had hoped, to model their hard-won skills of patience, discipline, and self-restraint, we had not bargained for the unsettling recognition they felt upon being confronted with their younger, wilder selves. "The little kids are *emo!*" they complained, using a popular slang term for visible performances of emotional dysregulation. They worried incessantly about whether the kids would hurt them during games and whether the kids would ever grow up and learn how to act properly. They got upset when we bent the game rules for the younger campers and were astonished to discover that we had bent the rules for them too. Along with the sense of commonality and connection built at the camp, then, came the uncomfortable feeling of recognizing one's own vulnerabilities, those managed at great personal cost, running free in someone else.

The new campers were certainly a handful. Gunnar was a little roly-poly kid with a long red ponytail and a short temper. He ran out of the room howling if anyone touched him when he wasn't expecting it, slamming the door behind him; he also liked to jump on people unexpectedly, to see what they would do. If someone got upset because of something he did, he would run out of the room and slam the door, overwhelmed by shame. If anyone spelled his name wrong, he would fly into a rage; if it wasn't corrected just right, he turned redder and redder until he hit the crisis point of giving up—"Never *mind!!!*"—at which point he would run out of the room and slam the door. The doors in the Unity Center were getting slammed a lot.

Danny, too, was extraordinarily sensitive to perceived slights. He hated curse words and what he called "Unkind Language." He also liked to sing, breaking spontaneously into a joyous hum that sometimes provoked Unkind Language from Gunnar and other campers who were hypersensitive to sound. He had an easier time when he was by himself, drawing photo-realistically detailed illustrations of characters from *Thomas the Tank Engine*. If a single freckle on Rosie the Engine's freckled face wound up out of place, however, he would crumple the paper into a ball. "I messed it up. I'm a failure. I always fail at everything." When he got stressed out, he and I would go for walks together, and he would tell me stories. "Now I would like to tell you a story about Rosie, the copycat friend of Thomas," he announced to me sweetly one day as we were on a walk together. All was going well, as I listened in silence to his memorized recitation of a story from the show, until I interrupted to ask him a question about "the trains" and how they work. "*Engines! They are **engines**!*" he corrected me in an agonized roar. A story developed through attention to the local relationships between details is easily destabilized by the participation of an unwittingly clumsy co-teller. Walking with him felt like walking on eggshells that could be broken merely by my being my separate self.

Instead, many of the Aspie campers remained focused on their own preoccupations, to the extent that it made it difficult for them to collaborate with others. Andrew Yollen had a quality like a lanky teenage puppy, all long legs and unstoppable enthusiasm. Elise told me he had saved up his own money to pay for an entire summer at the camp, no mean feat for a teenager with a developmental disability in a town where money was not abundant. He'd also saved up to buy a sword that Michael was designing and building for him. The first time Michael joined us at the Aspie Camp, Andrew bounded up to him. "Hello, what's-your-name. Do you know when my sword is going to be ready? Get a move on, on that." He asked me about his sword a lot, too, even though I didn't have access to any information about it. He interrupted everybody, often, sometimes in a wacky accent. The accent came from a character he'd played in his first weeks as a camper and had gotten pretty attached to. He was driving everybody crazy.

"He just can't recognize when there's another topic happening," William sighed, frustrated. "He's always off-topic. And I don't know how to teach him that." As a CIT, Andrew was supposed to be helping William out with building the props and the sets for our game. He really, really wanted to be helpful, and William really, really wanted to help him be helpful. But every time he came into the prop room, he wound up just talking about his own swords rather than helping with other people's. He kept announcing that he was going to carry short swords for our Capture the Flag games, even though we kept telling him that players could only use long swords because those were the only ones the whole group had practiced using. He had an idea for the design on his sword—could they make that for him? With Andrew helping, William could barely get any work done making props for anybody. It felt as though we were battling some sort of giant magnet, and its draw on Andrew's attention was stronger than anything we had to offer. Battling the magnet, day after day, was wearying.

The Theory of Extreme Awesomeness Ratio

By the last week, everyone was starting to fray around the edges. I often ran into Annie standing outside her office, looking pale and frazzled. For one thing, the campers liked to run into her office on rainy days, taking over her computer to draw their characters and print them out. But she felt shut out in other ways too. As a volunteer staffer and the parent of a program participant, her official role at the center was ambiguous, and she didn't always feel listened to. She had been trying for a while to raise concerns about the degree of physical affection she was seeing between Imogen and two of the CITs, Burke and Leo—they had recently discovered the fun of clustering up into a big snuggly pile and spent a lot of time sitting on each other, to the exclusion of the rest of the world—but she didn't feel like those concerns had been heard. And she felt that she had no access to Elise, who kept getting pulled into tense, closed-door meetings that Annie wasn't invited to.

"Did Elise tell you she has no memory?" she asked me one day after I'd found her in the hallway, shaking, and pulled her into a side room to ask if she was OK. "She scored a zero on those memory tests. I'm supposed to be her memory, but I can't be if nobody tells me things." Annie gave me a grim look. "I wonder if we are even going to get this thing off the ground."

I'd been wondering the same thing. Looking through the folder of media clippings the Unity Center had collected, I noticed that they all talked about how great the center was, but also about how hard it had been for the center to get the kind of grant funding it needed to open up its planned school or even to continue offering the services it currently offered. Various fund-raising schemes kept getting suggested, but none of them seemed to be taking hold.

Elise, battling to save the beleaguered Unity Center, worked hard to translate our adventures with the Journeyfolk into the kind of language that would be compelling to funding organizations, as well as to the public school district. These were important sources of potential financial viability, as the district could cover the tuition for a student's participation in Unity Center programming if it were considered a necessary component of their official education plan. After each day, we were supposed to go over our lesson plan, in which the Journeyfolk's practices had been translated into special education lingo, and evaluate whether we had met our goals and objectives for that day. I liked this ritual—it gave us a rare moment or two to catch our breath and reflect—but it never seemed to have all that much to do with what we were actually doing.

The last day of camp, after the monsters had been vanquished and the slain heroes mourned, after the campers had said their final good-byes and the CITs had gone off to see a movie together, as we put away the last of the props and tried not to wilt in the 90-plus-degree heat, Elise brought out a document for us to go over together: a statewide, standardized list of quality indicators for autism services that we could use to evaluate our programming. We struggled to come up with numbers from 0 to 3 expressing the extent to which we felt there was evidence for each particular quality indicator.[6] Were our evaluation reports (*What evaluation reports?*) written in a meaningful, understandable way? (*Meaningful to whom?*) Did our curriculum focus on maximizing independent functioning? (*What about interdependent functioning?*) These all seemed like decent ideas, but relating them to the work we were doing was not a straightforward process.

Our most exciting indicators of therapeutic progress, for example, tended to involve things like orcs. In our final game, rather than joining the rest of the CITs in the Monster Army, Andrew had insisted on reprising a character he'd played in one of our earlier games (the one with the wacky accent). We'd let him get away with it. It felt like he just wasn't ready to let go of being a heroic PC and move on to being an SPC monster, as the other CITs had done. But, we warned him, he needed to be prepared for the possibility that his character could be slain in battle and that he would have to reincarnate as a monster in the Orc Army. (When characters are slain in-game, the players are usually given another character to "reincarnate" into so as to finish out the game; because the rest of the CITs were playing orcs, that would likely be the character Andrew was given.) In the days leading up to the game, Andrew had repeatedly told us that he didn't want his character to be slain. We better protect him, he said, because he didn't want to come back as an orc. We better stay close by him. We better heal him if he got hit. The day of the game, however, something remarkable happened. Andrew told us that he had picked out his orc costume. If he got slain, and if we needed him to come back as an orc, then an orc he would be.

All the CITs, in fact, had found their way to be good monsters in the end. By the last game, they had developed a shtick, dancing out from behind the rocks while singing

> We're the Monsters—
> The happy, happy, Monsters—
> OF ROCK!!!

Then they wildly played air guitar.

In our last CIT meeting, Burke, Leo, Imogen, and I talked about the differences between the older CITs and the younger campers—about what maturity meant, and about their own growth as staff.[7] We went over the things that staff had to do: get along with other people, cultivate skills, deal with unexpected stuff that comes up. We all felt that they'd gotten a lot better at it over the past 2 weeks. When I asked what had helped them the most in that process, they told me that our meetings had helped—but even more important had been their friendship with each other.

"To be very scientific about it," Leo joked, "I call it the Theory of Extreme Awesomeness Ratio." When the awesomeness of one was low, the awesomeness of the others could help compensate for it. We ended the meeting with a cheer: *Theory of Extreme Awesomeness Ratio!*

"This has been the best 2 weeks of Sylvester's life," Annie told us in our last staff meeting. "Nobody's made fun of him, people have enjoyed him for just who he is."

"It's been the best 4 weeks of mine," Burke replied.

A few months later, I went to interview Leo on the campus of the local college where he had just started classes, hoping to pursue a career in psychology. I asked him how he felt that Asperger's had affected him.

"I think it's affected my life in many, many ways," he told me. "First, it started out negatively, because at first I felt very estranged, and very unusual. And then, it started to become a thing that made me part of something. Which—all that *anyone* wants is to be part—is to belong, somewhere. So, while it started negatively, in me feeling very separated and very wrong—I became part—part of a group, and part of a society, part of *people*."

For the Journeyfolk, to grow is to learn to tolerate being with our- selves and with each other in the completeness of our potentialities. It is a willingness to die and be reborn as something different and strange, to rock out amongst the monsters, to face that beast at the end of all things, and to recognize him within ourselves. At the camp, the continuities between the staff and the campers, the shared investment in cherished forms, practices and genre structures, and a deliberate ethos of accep- tance created a space where deep risks could be taken and where we could all experiment with new ways of being in the world.

To Dream of Heaven

Once the Summer of Adventure was over, I stayed in Brookfield to con- tinue my dissertation research and stayed in touch with many of the campers as I did so. I had the chance to interview many of them, a few of them multiple times. They were very polite, and did their best to give me good answers to my interview questions about Asperger's syndrome and how they felt about their diagnoses and so on. But what they really wanted to know, what they asked me about over and over again, was, *When are we going to do the camp again?* I didn't know what to tell them. I still don't.

"Institutional mourning," writes sociologist and comic book writer Eve Ewing (2018) in *Ghosts in the Schoolyard*, her book on Chicago school closings, "is the social and emotional experience undergone by individuals and communities facing the loss of a shared institution they are affiliated with—such as a school, church, residence, neighborhood, or business district—especially when those individuals or communities occupy a socially marginalized status that amplifies their reliance on the institution or its significance in their lives" (p. 127). As much as we may take with us—new strengths and sets of skills, new understandings of the bravery we are capable of—there is also that which lies beyond us, lost when a community is lost. When we lose such a place, we also lose the web of connections and shared histories that it holds. And we lose a version of ourselves—the person who we were in that community, our roles and relationships that existed only there.

In her ethnographic study of summer camps for children with chronic illness, Cindy Dell Clark (2003) describes a process she calls "imaginal coping"—"a socially situated and symbolically mediated activity that addresses issues of problematic meaning" (p. 95) through imaginative practices, including play, ritual, story, humor, and prayer. The kinds of summer camps she studied have often been found to improve the health outcomes of participants; the common assumption has been that this improvement results from didactics where kids learn biomedical information and approved techniques for self-care. But far more transformative, she suggests, is the "camp's shared idioculture" where "children participated in joint play-like activities that reconstructed meanings not through didactic information alone, but largely through play" (p. 100). Kids with diabetes paint with syringes; kids with asthma invent techniques for playing the noise-making spacer devices on their inhalers with their noses. Through this symbolic reconstruction of meaning, they transform the meaning of their difference as well, from a source of isolation and estrangement to a source of commonality and community with others. At the Aspie Camp, and through the Unity Center community more broadly, the meanings of Asperger's syndrome were transformed. At the camp, a condition that had been the source of alienation became an opportunity to be "a part of *people*," with all the new challenges that come with that.

The Journeyfolk know that story matters, and that certain stories grow best in certain worlds. Through story, we represent the deep intangibles of our experience, by organizing abstractions into sets of relationships connected by presuppositions about what kinds of relationships make sense. These presuppositions are deeply grounded in particular practical and interpretive contexts. In what follows, I talk about the stories we tell about autism, the way those stories relate to one another, and the way our stories help to shape us into the people we are. Because it is an ethnography, this book also focuses on the ways these stories take form in particular places and times: from a classroom in a school district with a history of creativity and contention around autism services and education to a support group whose members struggle to thrive under chaotic socioeconomic conditions to a clinic attempting to cultivate generalizable social skills within a medical school prioritizing the containment of contagious disease entities. Each of these settings support certain stories, with certain sets of assumptions: about what makes for trouble, about how selves are constituted, about how change happens, about which elements can comfortably coexist and which are mutually exclusive. Each of these settings thus creates a different sense of what is possible.

After Dream defeats Choronion at the Oldest Game and recovers his helmet, he attempts to leave the Kingdom of Hell (Gaiman, 1989). But Lucifer stops him. *Tell us why we should let you leave,* he asks. *Helmet or no, you have no power here—what power have dreams in Hell?*

You say I have no power? Dream replies. *Perhaps you speak truly. But—you say that dreams have no power here?*

Tell me, Lucifer Morningstar. . . .

Ask yourselves, all of you . . .

What power would Hell have if those imprisoned here were not able to dream of Heaven? (p. 22).

He walks out, and this time, they do not stop him.

2

Searching for a Place

Every Day Is a New Nightmare

By the end of the summer, Elise had confirmed what we had all begun to suspect: The Unity Center had not been able to secure the funds it needed to open the Unity School in the fall. Without the school in place, the center's ability to remain open as a community center was in jeopardy. Even with Annie filling many administrative roles on a volunteer basis, the organization would run out of money in a few months.

We hatched a number of frantic last-minute schemes: Push parents to do more fund-raisers? Apply for more funds from local foundations? Partner with other autism programs in the area? None of these initiatives were able to get traction. Our meetings started to focus on how to "close with dignity." Elise, frustrated and discouraged, started looking for other work. The families who had hoped to enroll their students there started to investigate other schooling options. And Annie, Sylvester, and I began to panic.

I'd moved into a small, smelly apartment in Brookfield, the region that housed the Unity Center, and signed a lease with the intention of spending the next 6 months there conducting an ethnography of the Unity School. My boyfriend had sublet his Chicago apartment and was getting ready to join me. On the way back from a trip home to see my parents at the end of August, the car I'd owned for 10 years that had carried my belongings all summer finally kicked the bucket. When I got back to Brookfield, in the large, banana-colored rental car I was driving around to every used-car lot in the region, Elise sat down with me and went over a list of other schools in the district that had programs for youth on the autism spectrum, including the names of some potential contacts. I called a bunch of people and left a bunch of messages. Then I called Annie.

Things were not going so well there either. The school year had started, but Sylvester was not in school. "The district made a terribly inappropriate placement recommendation," Annie told me. In the background, I heard Sylvester saying something anxiously that I couldn't quite hear. Annie sighed. "He likes to swing things around like swords in the apartment, and we have tiled ceilings. He just put a hole in the ceiling." A moment later: "Sylvester, I don't want to hug you right now; I'm on the phone." A moment later: "Oh, don't go off in a huff. No, that's enough. You can't pretend to hurt yourself. That's not OK."

I asked her what the school district had recommended. "They want to put him into an ILP with kids with multiple disabilities, with no other autistic kids. They have a padded time-out room. I'm trying to fight that."

"What's an ILP?" I asked her.

"Intensive Learning Program. It's a code name for kids with behavior disorders, kids who are in and out of psychiatric hospitalizations. And those kids do need programs—but I think those padded time-out rooms should be made illegal. We've been finding out that people have been dying because of these interventions." Indeed, just that morning I had read an article, circulated on a local autism-related e-mail list, about people on the autism spectrum who had died after being restrained by insufficiently trained personnel.

"Are you thinking about homeschooling?" I asked her. I knew a lot of parents, frustrated with the available school options, who had opted at least temporarily for do-it-yourself education.

"We're thinking about avoiding it at all costs," she sighed. "It's a total last resort. Neither of us will get what we need that way. Sylvester wants to be with his peers."

What they wanted, Annie told me, was for Sylvester to attend Valley View, a private school for middle and high school students on the autism spectrum that had opened a few years ago in Brookfield. They would need substantial assistance with tuition, but a number of local families had been able to make such arrangements. Since the announcement of the Unity Center closing, Annie told me, the school had been inundated with applications. But she had hope that Sylvester might be able to get a spot since they knew him there—he had participated in a number of their field trips and community activities.

"And I feel so bad for you," Annie continued ruefully. Annie liked anthropology, and she knew all about my dissertation project and its current uncertainties. I told her that with Elise's guidance, I was approaching a number of other schools in the region, including Valley View, and that I was also hoping to follow a few families who had been involved with the Unity Center, hang out with them, and observe their day-to-day lives and daily routines as they figured out their next steps. Would she and Sylvester be interested?

"We don't really have any *routines*," she warned me. "We just do what we do. Every day is a new nightmare." She laughed. "Just kidding." Paused. "Sort of."

After a bit more discussion, Annie said I could hang around with them as they did their thing. "When do you want to schedule your next . . . appointment?" she asked, casting around for a word for whatever it was I was going to be doing with them. We settled on that coming Monday.

And so it was that I spent the next 6 months of my ethnographic fieldwork following kids through the labyrinth of their school system, as they, their families, and school administrators tried to figure out where they belonged. It was not a straightforward process. The students were a very diverse bunch, and the one thing they all had in common was how hard it was for them to find and maintain a place for themselves in the world. Swinging between extremes of rage and withdrawal, hyper-focused attention and disinterest, passionate commitment and disengagement, their ongoing, chronic dysregulation left them reliant on their environment for organization, order, and stability. They worked to create that stability in a variety of ways: through resisting change, through prioritizing hobbies that allowed them to create and work with predictable systems, through slowly building elaborate networks of in-jokes with peers, through retreating from chaotic social interactions into passive withdrawal or active fantasy lives. In the world outside their control, however, these attempts were often uprooted, as they were moved from classroom to classroom, program to program, in and out of formal schooling. They were constantly confronted with disruption, discontinuity, and fragmentation— their social relationships tenuous, their ability to remain anywhere perpetually threatened by the explosions they catalyzed. The result was a worsening cycle of volatility and social estrangement.

The Aspie kids of Brookfield were caught up in what sociologists Ul-rich Beck and Elisabeth Beck-Gernsheim (2002) refer to as "institution-alized individualism": Many aspects of their lives were shaped by large, geographically dispersed bureaucracies that compelled them to think of themselves as decontextualized individuals on their own personalized life-path. Meanwhile, opportunities to feel embedded within consistent, secure sets of social ties were increasingly eroded by ubiquitous require-ments that they move within such systems in such a way. Individual-ized assessment and "individualized education plans" (IEPs) claimed to depict and address their particular needs in the education system, but these amalgamations of scores and recommendations, as well as their consequences, were dictated by a system way larger than any individual child and his or her world. By law, they were entitled to a "free and ap-propriate" education through the public school system; what that means in practice was extraordinarily complex and contested. School districts offered some educational options (classrooms characterized by their mix of students, approach to curriculum, goals for student outcomes, and teaching staff; services that students would be pulled out of class for such as speech therapy; and accommodations and supports such as an in-class aide) but not others. Health insurance plans covered some services but not others, under some circumstances but not others; out-of-pocket costs and availability of services varied widely. Families were thus confronted by a lot of choices but were also operating within a lot of constraints, many of which seemed mysterious and arcane, and all of which were regulated by large and inscrutable bureaucracies represented by people who were often frustrated and frustrating.

Beck (2002) describes the lives produced within contemporary in-dividualizing institutions as "tightrope biographies": "Everyone is in constant danger of falling to the ground but attempts, with greater or less artistic skill and awareness, to get control of their own life: a few are very lucky, many others less so" (p. 52). The pictures this work draws of the types of citizens produced by this system are those who can more or less hang on within it: "the actors, builders, jugglers, stage managers of their own biographies and identities and also of their social links and networks" (Beck & Beck-Gernsheim, 2002, p. 23). But it is those who do not function so effectively as flexible, adaptive self-regulators who often become the most deeply embroiled within bureaucratic systems of governance: the special education system, the penal system, and the "institutional circuit" (Hopper, Jost, Hay, Welber, & Haugland, 1997) of jails, shelters, and supported housing. And thus, they are the ones most deeply shaped by its combination of standardization and atomization.

The vulnerabilities displayed by the Aspie kids developed and deepened in such ongoing interactions with their particular social environments. Through their experiences in the school system, they learned that how you learn determines where you belong—and very often, what they learned is that they don't belong anywhere. Too volatile or too easily overwhelmed to learn in mainstream classrooms, too book smart for the classrooms for kids with global cognitive impairments, too wordy for the classrooms for kids with communication impairments, and too disorganized to complete the work of gifted programs, they bounced from setting to setting. They fell farther and farther behind, both academically and in their scrupulously measured socio-emotional development. And they became more and more deeply estranged from the coordinated give-and-take of sustained sociality, developing instead a brittle, explosive emotional style and a deep distrust for the system that was supposed to be nurturing them.

For a number of these students, the Asperger's syndrome diagnosis became a refuge. A new kind of classification, it provided a wider view of who they were: their strengths as well as their weaknesses, their history as well as their current struggles. And it offered an invitation into a shared culture characterized by an ethos of creativity and an ethic of inventive repair, a rebuilding of broken connections both material and social. Through this process, students diagnosed with Asperger's syndrome learned to identify deeply with their diagnosis—and with its position at the expanding edges of the stigmatized category of "developmental disability." In the process of learning who they are, they also learn who they are not: Their condition is frequently defined *against* classifications such as "behavior disorder" or "emotional disturbance," understood to fall under the domain of mental health rather than developmental disability.

In the chapters that follow, this book charts the various arenas in which this expansion of the category of neurodevelopmental disability into new arenas of sociality and interaction is taking place, its origins, and its consequences. We follow its looping path through science policy and research into support groups, clinics, and schools; its uptake within families; and its transformation through creative play and subcultural folk mythologies. Neurodevelopmental diagnostic knowledge develops, percolates through worlds beyond the lab and the clinic, and becomes a prominent part of the organization of identities and social lives in places where the meanings of these conditions get negotiated and deployed in consequential ways. That knowledge is shaped through the particularities of such places, where people affected by autism spectrum conditions— not only those diagnosed but also those who surround them who may also share many of these propensities themselves—come together to learn and play, to fight and yell and freak out and repeat things, to coordinate and create, to build and to break and to rebuild again.

We'll Fix Her Up Real Good, Don't Worry

A few days after my conversation with Annie, I get permission from the school director to stop by Valley View. The school is housed in a church, in a well-to-do neighborhood; the walls are covered with pictures of little children and little lambs and encouragement to memorize the Lord's Prayer. I wander into the building and am greeted by a tall young man who introduces himself rather formally as Roland. I explain that I'm there to see Kirk, the head of the school. He nods and offers to take me to him, as that is, fortunately, the very direction in which he is currently headed. Roland, I come to discover, is a junior at Valley View, and he always talks like that.

Roland takes me to a darkened classroom where Kirk and a bunch of big teenage boys are sitting around a table on chairs that all look too small. The younger kids are in another classroom with Stan, the other teacher. One of the older students, Darren, is working on fixing a broken computer. The others are trying to have a discussion about *The Witch of Blackbird Pond* (Speare, 1958), but things keep getting off-track, hopelessly so once I show up. I tell them I'm doing a research project on Asperger's syndrome.

"That's easy," Kieran cuts in, cheerfully. He's a big guy with a mop of curls who looks much older than his 14 years. Everyone seems to be watching him nervously. "There's no such thing. The category is bullshit. It's way too broad, basically. Anyone can have Asperger's, basically, the way it's written. So it's totally meaningless. Now, *autism*," he continues, "autism is a real thing. If you can't talk, if you're completely fucked up, basically. But Asperger's is nothing. It's not some kind of a *disease*."

"It's a mental *disorder*," Roland sighs.

Kirk tries a few more times to get us focused back on *The Witch of Blackbird Pond* but eventually gives up and tells a long, intermittently very funny story about his recent trip to Aruba.

Valley View teaches kids all the usual subjects—math, science, literature, social studies, a smattering of languages—but at the heart of the curriculum are group projects and the ongoing work of coordinating ourselves around them. Sometimes, these projects are as simple as a coherent conversation, a running joke, an afternoon where nobody has a meltdown and everybody stays in the room. Much of the time, the projects are more concrete. Just before I arrived, the students had worked together to build a very impressive treehouse that they used for sleepover parties and other special events. In the back of one of the classrooms was a massive marble maze, built by the students, that spelled out "Asperger's Can Be Fun!" It was covered with items that represented quirky geniuses who might have had Asperger's: a chessboard for Bobby Fischer, records for Thomas Edison. Darren had wired it so that the word *fun!* lit up when the marble hit it. Next to that was a giant wooden replica of Andy Warhol's Campbell's Soup can, a reference to the idea that Warhol's work, with its repetitive variations on a single pop-culture fascination, had a distinctly Aspie quality. My first week at Valley View, we worked together on creating a haunted house featuring a Mad Scientist's Lab. "We're going to paint it all whacko," Kirk explained. "I got the most awful colors I could find."

The school encouraged an ethos of experimentation, tinkering, and creativity. We spent a good bit of time, later that year, brainstorming and building innovative mousetraps, inspired by the saying *Build a better mousetrap and the world will beat a path to your door.* Morning lessons from Kirk would often be full of long stories of "wacky" people he knew who had unusual lives, unconventional careers. "The world needs more inventors," Kirk was fond of saying to the students. "I want you all thinking like [Thomas] Edisons. We need more inventions. There have been a lot of inventors with Asperger's."

Things were constantly being fixed up at Valley View. Kieran loved to work on 8-track machines, buying them broken and then tweaking the wiring until sound flooded warmly out of the speakers. "They love their junk," Kirk sighed, rolling his eyes to heaven as he unloaded another box of duct tape and old computer parts out of the car and into the students' waiting hands. The same ethic of appreciative rehabilitation was extended to the students. Sitting in the classroom, I along with everyone else could often hear Kirk in the back of the room, talking on the phone to some desperate parent. "The district really messed her up, huh? We're going to fix her up. We'll fix her up real good, don't worry."

Kirk ran Valley View on a shoestring budget, and those strings, metaphorically speaking, often came out of his own shoes: He paid many of the school's expenses out of pocket while waiting for tuition payments that had often been reduced for low-income families or tangled up in lengthy and uncertain legal battles with school districts. The teachers in the school volunteered or worked at near-minimum wage. It often felt like they all kept Valley View afloat as a labor of love, a kind of sanctuary for kids who didn't fit in anywhere else and who had gotten mangled badly as a result.

We Had a Whole New Kid

Allen, an 11-year-old in the younger kids' classroom, was one of those kids. A sulky skateboarder, dramatically tall for his age, Allen had always been intense in his temperament and sensitivities. As a baby, he was fussy and difficult to soothe. As he got older, he was slow to learn to speak. In kindergarten, he became so overwrought when frustrated that he would bang his head against the table. The small private school he was attending told his mother, Corinne, that he couldn't come back for first grade. "They didn't feel that they could address whatever was [going on]," she told me. "They didn't want him, and I didn't want to force him to be somewhere where he wasn't wanted." So Allen started public school in first grade, "in a typical, mainstream, classroom, about 28 kids with one teacher, and it was disastrous. He was hiding under tables, not doing work, running out of the classroom. And that initiated us into the special education arena." Corinne started doing research on the Internet, typing in terms like *explosive child* and following where they led. It led her to OASIS, one of the major information sites available at that time about Asperger's. "Wow," Corinne said to herself, "that sounds like my kid." She was especially intrigued by the idea of sensory integration dysfunction: that Allen's acting-out and withdrawal might be caused, in part, by a difference in how his brain processed sensory input. She took him to be evaluated by a series of developmental pediatricians, and he was diagnosed first with PDD-NOS, and then with Asperger's.

The family moved to a new school district, and Allen started second grade in an "inclusion class": two special education teachers and an aide, in a class that contains both kids who are and kids who are not receiving special education services. He thrived. "It was a wonderful, excellent, dream-come-true year, compared to what first grade was. It had everything to do with the teachers—they did a lot of remediation with him. He came out of his shell a bit more, he gained more confidence in himself in that classroom, he was highly supported emotionally, socially—just, all around, great environment for him." He made friends for the first time; he participated in school assemblies. The next year, for third grade, he stayed in the same kind of program—but he had new teachers. And everything changed. "By the end of the first semester of that year it started to become clear that it wasn't the appropriate place for him. The schoolwork was getting harder; his frustration levels were skyrocketing; the teachers didn't really want to know anything about anything. *He was a bad kid* is the message that I got." Allen started injuring himself in class again: banging his head, scratching himself, pinching himself. He was put on a behavior plan where he was sent out into the hallway if he misbehaved; he would sit there alone for hours. By the end of his third-grade year, he told his therapist that he was thinking about stabbing himself. "It was devastating, devastating. And it all revolved around school, and his image of himself from school, and the low self-esteem, and the: *[I'm] stupid, I can't do anything right, I'm never gonna learn anything. That kind of thing.*" At the recommendation of the therapist, his family advocated for him to be switched to another classroom.

However, the only placement made available to him within his school district was a classroom for children with communication impairments. Allen was the only child in the class who could fluently speak. "He was the highest-functioning child. The reason I thought it was worth trying was because I was very, very impressed with the teacher in the classroom. And the idea was to have him gain some self-worth, some trust in school again, to just let it be a kind of no-brainer, stress-free end of the school year. And it helped. However, he knew—he was—he didn't belong in that classroom. And it still didn't do the greatest things for his self-esteem." The school district wanted Allen to stay in that classroom for fourth grade. Two weeks into his fourth-grade year, he started refusing to go on the school bus. "He was diagnosed at that time with severe anxiety disorder, depression, suicidal ideation. It was too much. The pressure was just, just too much. And so I took him *out*."

Corinne homeschooled Allen while looking for other options. Then she found Valley View, and everything turned around:

> He's started to believe in himself again, trust in himself, he started trusting teachers, he gained confidence in his academic ability. There was no homework, so there wasn't any pressure at home—and so there wasn't that head-butting, at home. He just started to lose some of the anxiety, from the public school, feeling like everybody was staring at him because he was having difficulty. By the end of that year, he said—it was so funny, the way he said it: *I'm with people that get me,* I think is what he said. Something like that. He was—he was happy. He was just—he was a happy kid. And so now we're on our third year there, and he's confident, he has friends, he has things he does, he's—you know, we still have issues, but so does everybody.

For the first time, at Valley View, Allen had a best friend: Jerome, another floppy-haired kid in his class. "When I met Jerome," Allen told me, "we were right away, like, *wanna be friends*? He and I, we're, like, the same. I taught him how to be like me, and stuff. I taught him how to be cool, how to joke around and stuff. He's like my brother. I taught him how to be the same. We're the same, basically. My other friends, they wouldn't know how to mess around. I used to be in a class with . . ." He shook his head, stared into the distance. "Kids who—pick their nose in class, and stuff. I didn't use to connect with any of my friends. They used to pick on me . . ."

"He started [Valley View] by November of his fourth-grade year," Corinne told me. "And we had a whole new kid after a few months. I could show you a neuropsych [neuropsychological evaluation] from before he went there and a neuropsych from after he went there, and if there weren't names, on that, you would think you were reading two different child's descriptions."

To understand what's so significant about what Corinne is saying here, it is helpful to know a bit about "neuropsychs"—what they are, what they do. A "neuropsych," or neuropsychological evaluation, consists largely of a series of tests, usually alongside an interview with the test subject and perhaps with their family members. The subject's performance on these tasks guides inferences about their underlying brain function and, in particular, the potential presence of brain illness or injury. Developed after the First World War created a generation of battle survivors who suffered from lingering damage to localized brain areas, neuropsychological evaluations are now commonly given to assess cognitive changes in the elderly as well as learning disabilities in children, and are frequently administered as part of the process of being diagnosed with a neurodevelopmental disorder such as autism spectrum disorder. They assess a range of traits that characterize a subject's approach to the world: perception, learning, memory, attention, cognition. However, the concept of the brain lesion still metaphorically organizes the representations of the phenomena that have replaced it as objects of investigation. Although what is being investigated is now understood as a systemic phenomenon involving entire processing systems—whole-brain regions and the connections between them—the underlying model persists even as it is applied in new contexts and to new targets. The goal is still to infer the presence of some discrete problem in the brain that manifests through differences from the norm in task performance. Some of these characteristics are presumed to be more or less stable over time while others are presumed to change due to illness or healing processes, but all are assumed to be inherent to the individual being evaluated. The presupposition is that the tests locate bodily pathologies of the individual test subject. Thus, the change in Allen's neuropsychological profile, between who he was in a stressful environment and who he was in a welcoming one, is remarkable to Corinne: the same kid is not supposed to have two such different reports.

But looked at in another way, it makes sense. All the phenomena brought together through such testing—perception, attention, learning, memory, and so forth—share a distinguishing feature: By definition, each always has some kind of an object. Learning is always the learning *of* particular material. Perception is always the perception *of* a particular stimulus. Memory is always the memory *of* particular content. That second term—the thing that is learned, perceived, remembered—is an intrinsic element of the phenomenon being assessed. Taking place at the interface where self meets world, neuropsychological evaluations are all about our encounter with *something else*. Neuropsychological formulations, as they are currently configured, thus provide an opportunity to dwell in the contingent—contingent in the sense of both its initial etymology of "to touch with" and in the sense of dependence on circumstance. They are stories of how we touch and are touched by the world around us. But they are often not used in that way.

While neuropsychological formulations intrinsically evoke and involve material outside of the perceiving, learning, remembering body, these phenomena are often then reconceptualized exclusively as properties of decontextualized, singular brains. This process does a particular kind of interpretive transformation work, by reinscribing the environment, that always-present second term, as a feature of the bodily properties of the child. It is a dual process of expansion and constriction in which the explicitly extrasomatic is evoked and then obscured. Through this process, the world of the child becomes localized within that child's body, justifying their removal from a network of existing interpersonal connections to place them according to their measured impairments.

For Allen, how well he's doing has a lot to do with his relationships with the people around him—a teacher who clicks with him, friends who know him, people who *get* him (or don't). But these relationships are often transformed into resources to be transactionally exchanged based on individual characteristics inferred and quantified. (Burke described the process to me one day when we were sitting around talking: "So then in sixth grade, when they said I was autistic, all of a sudden, I showed up in school, and I had an aide! O-*kaaaay*. And then, in eighth grade, they decided I didn't need the aide anymore, and they took the aide away. What?!") These students are embroiled in a highly bureaucratized system that simultaneously atomizes and aggregates them. It is a system that is supposed to help and support kids but with which they, and their families, are frequently in fierce conflict—a conflict I saw close-up as I watched Annie and Sylvester negotiate his IEP.

You Ripped Apart My IEP

My heart was pounding with nervousness as I rang the doorbell for my first ethnographic visit. But when Sylvester answered the door, let out a yell of joy, and threw his arms around me, I was instantly cheered. By the time I'd gotten up the stairs to their apartment, he was already telling me about the new sword he was going to get for his birthday party, which Annie was throwing for him next week in collaboration with a few Journeyfolk. He had decided that the game we would play would be a combination of Journeyfolk and the cartoon show *Naruto*, well loved among Sylvester's peers, based on a Japanese manga comic about a team of young ninjas in training. He'd learned lots of "jitsus" (he used the term to mean special battle moves from a card game he liked, also about ninjas) and had made some up, too, for us to use at the "Journaruto" birthday party. He demonstrated them for me, rapid-fire. They all consisted of an elemental battle-cry—"Thunderstrike!"—and a hand gesture, accompanied by an intense expression and followed by an explanation of their effect, which I could never quite make sense of.

While I was hanging out with Sylvester, Annie made us a quesadilla—she showed me how to do it, laughing about *anthropology*—and made a slew of phone calls: to Sylvester's educational advocate; to doctors, asking about test results; to Elise, telling her she wouldn't be able to keep volunteering at the Unity Center until Sylvester's school situation was sorted out. Her big project for the afternoon, however, was typing up a letter that needed to be dropped off at the Brookfield School District office that afternoon. Sylvester had a meeting coming up, to discuss his IEP. This was the meeting where a team of educators and administrators would decide, with some amount of input from him and Annie, what his learning needs were, and what classroom would best suit his needs. This is a complex and often (as was the case for Sylvester) deeply contested process.

In the United States, eligibility for special education services is governed by legislation initially passed in 1990 (as the Individuals with Disabilities Education Act, or IDEA) as an update of the 1975 Education for All Handicapped Children Act, and reauthorized in 2004 as the Individuals with Disabilities Education Improvement Act. Under these laws, every child in the United States is entitled to a free and appropriate public education. What this means in practice for each student, within a highly standardized system populated by idiosyncratic youth, is mediated by a document called the IEP. Each student who is identified as having a disability that affects their learning is entitled to have such a plan and to have it be followed.

Although these documents vary between states and between school systems, federal regulations dictate a number of elements. The IEP must contain quantified assessments of the student's current level of functioning in areas that are related to their participation in the school's curriculum. These areas include the student's academic performance and various abilities related to learning; it may also include measures of their social and behavioral competence. It must also contain specific and measurable annual goals, broken down into short-term benchmarks, and must specify how progress will be measured. The IEP lists the special education services that are to be provided to the student, supports to be provided, and modifications, if any, to be made to standardized tests. It spells out the extent to which the student will be integrated with nondisabled peers and (for students 14 and older) the kinds of services that will be provided to help them transition out of the supports of the school system and into a more independent adulthood. Although these plans are supposedly "individualized," in practice, their design and implementation actually depend a great deal on what kinds of classroom groups and resources are available, which itself depends on funding decisions made at a variety of higher levels from the local to the federal.

The IEP is supposed to be negotiated collaboratively in recurring meetings including parents, teachers, school administrators, and often the student, along with others who know them. Sometimes, these meetings go smoothly; other times, they become contentious, as the various stakeholders involved disagree about what the student's needs and capacities are and how they are best served with the limited resources available. If disagreements cannot be resolved in the meeting, parents and school staff have the option of going to mediation; if this fails, the last resort is a "due process hearing." At a due process hearing, the disagreeing parties (often supported by lawyers) present their cases to a hearing officer who adjudicates the dispute. This is often colloquially referred to as "suing the district" or "going to litigation." A 2014 publication from the Center for Appropriate Dispute Resolution in Education, a program funded by the Office of Special Education Programs at the U.S.

Department of Education, notes: "Due process is considered the most adversarial, least collaborative dispute resolution option, and may damage the working relationship between educators and families" (p. 7). In many cases, however, by the time things reach this point, this working relationship is already significantly strained.

Such was the case for Annie and Sylvester, along with many of the other families I got to know in Brookfield. The letter that Annie was typing up, in anticipation of her upcoming IEP meeting, notified the school officials that Annie would be recording and transcribing everything that would be said at the meeting. By this point, Annie had come to take for granted that lies would be told and promises broken, and she wanted some way of maintaining accountability. Later that afternoon, she would drop the letter off at the school in person and receive documentation that it had been received; otherwise, she told me with a knowing look, "They will *lose* it." In case I had missed her nonverbal implication, she added, "In quotes."

These efforts notwithstanding, the meeting did not go well. I didn't attend—Annie figured that too many people were going to be there for her and Sylvester's comfort as it was—but when I asked her about it a few days later, she gave a shudder. "Well, we're going to due process," she sighed. So I went with her and Sylvester to meet with Dara, a local attorney who assisted parents needing legal advocacy with their school districts. I sat with them as Dara flipped through the IEP, throwing out a list of rapid-fire complaints, first in technical language about the difference between standardized scores and percentiles that Annie scribbled down frantically and then in some plain talk.

"Goals and objectives suck," Dara paraphrased. "Measurements suck. Scores aren't reported in a way I understand. Goals and objectives don't match each other, so they aren't measurable. The kid is suffering. Tell them they have 10 days to fix it. Then you're going to start spending their money."

"You really ripped apart that IEP," Annie said to her admiringly as we left. "I could see it shredding before my eyes."

Sylvester's face turned ferocious. He looked like he was about to throw a jitsu at Dara. "YOU RIPPED APART MY IEP!" he growled.

"Shhhh—it's OK—she is a *friend*," I reassured him solemnly, feeling myself slip into the formal speech of his fantasy world of sparring factions. It felt less strange than the world we were in, one where the plan intended to arrange a child's life to his benefit instead becomes the enemy.

The Widening Domain of Emperor Ner

In addition to Annie, a number of Brookfield parents were attempting to get the school district to pay for tuition at Valley View. To do so, they needed to demonstrate that the district had no options available that were appropriate for their Asperger's kids. However, Valley View was not the only school program in Brookfield dedicated to serving the needs of youth with Asperger's syndrome.

Following the closing of ASPIRE, the school district had opened two classrooms for younger and older teens diagnosed with Asperger's and similar autism spectrum conditions, a program I call ASPEN, located within a building dedicated to special education services. Sylvester was too young to attend ASPEN yet, but for older kids, demonstrating that the district had no appropriate schooling options meant proving that ASPEN was inadequate to meet their needs. Relations between ASPEN administrators and the community that had formed around Valley View were therefore pretty tense. Remarkably, however, the head of each program took pity on the stranded ethnographer and allowed me to observe in their classrooms and to interview the members of their school community—parents, students, and staff—who wished to participate in my project. I don't think I was ever able to fully assuage the worry of all members of each community that I was actually there as a spy for the other.

The vibe at ASPEN, at least on the surface, is very different from that of Valley View. Upon my arrival at the building, a modern-looking facility emblazoned with the logo of the Brookfield special education system (ACER), I check in at a front desk surrounded by plate glass. There's a sign declaring the school a Hat-Free Zone. I sign my name, write down what I'm there for, and get directions to the classroom and an ID badge to wear while I'm there. Every time I slow up my stride and start to look a little lost, a friendly adult stops me with a no-nonsense inquiry about where I'm going and what I'm up to. The adults are very clearly in charge here. The conversations and interactions in the hallways are almost all between adult professionals—when they are accompanied by a kid, the kid is usually silent. The students aren't really supposed to be spending much time in the hallways, anyway—they're liminal, transitional spaces.

Unlike at Valley View, where everyone is in everyone else's face all the time, here the students spend much of their time faced toward a row of computers. If Valley View encourages its students to become mad scientists, ASPEN encourages them to become computer scientists. The students work on the computers during work time and then stay on the computers during free time, playing games or making kooky art out of things they've found on the Internet. Nonetheless, unlike in the sterility of the hallways, in the classroom there's a flourishing kid culture. The banter between the students is nonstop, an ongoing balance of adversarial teasing (*I'm going to insult you*) and careful maintenance of group ties (*and you're going to get the in-joke I made while doing it*). A lot of the jokes are about scary things: velociraptors, pedophiles, the stigma of cognitive impairment. The teachers tolerate it, warily, to a point.

My first day in the room for older teens, I see a lot of familiar faces. Burke is there and is amazed to see me again. "Why are you a stalker?!" he asks. I try to explain that I'm not a stalker; I'm an ethnographer. He's not really supposed to be in the classroom either; he's already graduated and moved on to the vocational/technical program that is supposed to help him transition into the work world. But he comes back all the time to hang out anyway. The teachers allow this, when he behaves himself. Luke, a Journeyfolk camper whom I haven't seen since the summer, runs up and greets me with a few tales of World War II naval battles. "OK, bye!" he says when he's done and takes off. Zander, whom I haven't met before, is on the computer making greeting cards. "Sorry I Sent the Zombies to Your House! Happy Easter!" reads one of them, against the backdrop of a giant Christmas tree.

This kind of creative bricolage characterizes the classroom culture. Linguistic anthropologists Elinor Ochs and Olga Solomon (2008; see also Solomon, 2008) have identified a conversational technique often employed by people on the spectrum that they call "proximal relevance": participating in interactions by making a comment that is relevant to what has just been said based on structural algorithms grounded in shared objective knowledge rather than based on its relevance to the broader topic under consideration. At ASPEN, proximal relevance is elevated to a collective art form, and perhaps even a form of resistance to the teacher-determined concerns of the classroom context. We spend a lot of time disassembling discursive systems and tacking them back together in new and funny arrangements. On the chalkboard, there's an ever-changing Pie of the Day. (I've changed the name of the program, but its original name prominently featured the letters P–I–E). Today the Pie of the Day is Eskimo Pie. (Ethnic jokes are popular, despite the teachers' efforts to keep them to a minimum; a lot of the classroom humor revolves around deploying category terms whose meanings are multiple and contested, and juxtaposing those meanings in unexpected ways.) Another day, the Pie of the Day is Cutie Pie. Usually, the pies refer indirectly to something going on in the classroom. The week Zander got arrested, the Pie of the Day was Jailbird Pie.

Pie of the Day was Greg's idea, and he was usually the one responsible for coming up with new ones. He was the instigator of quite a lot of the creative material that circulated the classroom. His most famous piece, which he began one afternoon during a free-writing session and developed for some time after that, was "Jurassic Pie," a story in which everyone in the classroom was recast as battling dinosaurs. Emily, the tough, funny assistant teacher, was a ferocious beast. Cory, who napped all the time, was a sleepy-saur. Jurassic Pie was very popular, and I felt kind of sad that he didn't put me in it.

Greg hadn't always been at the center of things. In elementary school, according to his mother, he'd been isolated and lonely. The other kids threw balls at him on the playground; rather than throwing them back, he would go and lie down in the far corners of the playground where he could be easily overlooked. One time, she told me, a social worker actually stepped over him on her way out to the parking lot. By the end of fourth grade, he was refusing to go to school at all. His mother put him in a small private school and things got slightly better, but she still felt he needed more help than he was getting. He'd received a variety of tentative diagnoses—obsessive-compulsive disorder, attention-deficit/hyperactivity disorder, Tourette's syndrome—but none of them really seemed to fit. So he went through a series of neuropsychological evaluations and a consultation with a neurologist. She was surprised, at first, when Greg was diagnosed with Asperger's—his biggest issues, other than getting pushed around by other kids, were his lack of physical coordination and a tendency to get overwhelmed by sensory input, neither of which she had thought of as part of Asperger's until the neurologist told her otherwise. However, the diagnosis gave him access to the newly opening ASPIRE program, which had seemed like a good fit with its small size, well-trained staff, and rigorous academics.

At first, at ASPIRE, he struggled to make friends with the other kids. But with time, he found his way. "By the second year," his mother told me, "everything changed. Somehow, something clicked, and he was doing beautifully socially. Maybe he got used to the kids and the teachers. That's a big possibility. It just takes him that long to warm up. So that was good." But soon, the rug was pulled out from under him again, with the closing of ASPIRE. "Just before the Christmastime of his third year there, which was ninth grade, they sat all the parents down and said, *this program, Brookfield's not gonna pick it up for next year. It's closed . . .*"

Greg's mother and a number of the other ASPIRE parents got together and lobbied the school district to offer a similar program, dedicated to the particular needs and gifts of students with Asperger's syndrome, and ASPEN was the result. Like ASPIRE, the ASPEN curriculum encourages students to consider Asperger's syndrome as a complex condition bringing gifts and challenges. The day I arrived in Alice's classroom for older teens, the students were reading Daniel Tammet's (2006) *Born on a Blue Day: Inside the Mind of an Autistic Savant.* The book is an autobiography of a man on the autism spectrum whose ability to perceive numbers as beautiful colors assists him in performing astounding calculations. "Do you ever see numbers as beautiful?" Alice was asking a student as I came in. (He didn't.)

However, joining a program for students on the autism spectrum comes with a cost as well: the stigma of developmental disability. Kids like Greg, whose challenges are pretty subtle, often associate developmental disability with more pronounced impairments, and do a lot of interpretive work trying to figure out the extent to which this category applies to them.

"Why are we learning math with someone who's not a math teacher?" Greg grumbled one afternoon at ASPEN, during a math class that Alice was leading.

Alice thought about this for a moment. "I'm a special ed teacher," she replied. "So I know about *everything.*"

"Oh great," Greg replied. "We get the teacher for *nerrrrr.* That's great."

Ner, in the ASPEN classroom, was both a taunt (*nee-ner, nee-ner, neeee-ner*) and a slang term for cognitive impairment. The term played a central role in the teasing battles that made up a substantial part of the social conversations at ASPEN. Shortly after my arrival at ASPEN, the students proudly introduced me to Emperor Ner, a rather extraordinary piece of folk art they had meticulously crafted and now treated with great affection. Emperor Ner was a big sock puppet with a twisty mouth and many, many eyes—a design that, to me at least, suggested both heightened ability and freakish deviance.

The issue of the classroom's ambiguous *ner* status was still on Greg's mind later that day. "Why am I in a special ed class?" he asked Alice. "And what about your French class?" Alice also taught a French class that had kids from the entire school building, including those who weren't in ASPEN. "Everyone you teach except us isn't *ner ner.*"

Again, Alice gave this question a bit of consideration before answering. "You're very bright. You're here because this is a good place for you. You like it here." She assured him that he did not have intellectual disabilities. "You *are* diagnosed with Asperger's syndrome. Which is a nice thing to be diagnosed with because it's almost like a talent, rather than a disability." Then it was time for us to get back on task. "So prove your talent by solving this math problem."

Students like Greg, who can kinda sorta get along in mainstream classrooms, aren't really supposed to be in programs like ASPEN. Federal law dictates that students with disabilities must be educated in the "least restrictive environment"—and "restriction," although its legal meaning is ambiguous and contested, is, in practice, most often interpreted to mean as close as possible to a general education classroom, with nondisabled peers and without special supports or extra resources (Marx et al., 2014).[1] Only if a child cannot be successful in such a classroom can he or she be moved to a more "restrictive" environment. Greg, for example, had to return to his old school district and spend a single day demonstrating that he couldn't function in that environment (which he did by becoming so miserable that his mother could argue that he'd been traumatized) before he could be admitted to ASPIRE. The system is set up according to the presumption that the best environment for a kid is with typically developing peers and that every step away from that is a step in the wrong direction, a step toward an abnormality associated with failure and entailing the curtailment of individual freedom.

Programs like ASPIRE and ASPEN do not map well onto such a linear continuum. Their students were instead identified with a classification that's "almost like a talent, rather than a disability"—a classification that spoke to their strengths and interests as well as their weaknesses and vulnerabilities. The structures of the environment nurtured collaborative, co-regulated relationships between the students—even allowing Burke to hang around postgraduation as long as he didn't cause too much trouble—facilitated by the creative culture that emerges when a whole bunch of kids who think and interact with the world this way get to hang out together for a long time, their fragmentations recombined into appealing new forms.

Kids like Sylvester, who had experienced the fun of autistic community at the Unity Center, wanted to be part of a program like that, and their parents often wanted it for them too. But the question of who actually belongs in Asperger-specific programs was far from straightforward, given that the diagnosis of Asperger's syndrome was in constant, contested flux. Although Sylvester had come to strongly identify with his diagnosis, it was not immediately clear that there would be a place for him in the vision of Asperger's syndrome upheld by Valley View.

Can I Have a Half-Day?

Annie had written to the school district to inform them that she would be placing him at Valley View within 10 days; however, she hadn't yet gotten a clear answer from Kirk about whether he had been accepted. Sylvester had gone in for a day of testing with Kirk's wife, Uma. He had gaped at her living room library—"I read at grade level, so this is, like, heaven!"—and then had struggled through several hours of math problems and questions like *How are a fish and a submarine similar?* which were meant to measure his abstract and conceptual reasoning abilities. ("Both swim!" he sang jubilantly). He'd hung in there and stayed on task well enough to earn a trip to Pizza Hut, but Kirk remained concerned about Sylvester's impulsive behaviors, his meltdowns, the ways he seemed only barely in control of his body. Following the meeting, Kirk invited Sylvester to spend a day at Valley View to try it out but insisted that both Annie and I accompany him.

When I arrive that day, Roland has Kieran backed into a corner, finger in his face, speaking very intensely. "If you mess with Sylvester," he declaims in his warm, old-time radio announcer voice, "I WILL break every bone in your body."

"Who's Sylvester?" Kieran responds.

Roland is in the middle of trying to explain how he knows Sylvester from the Unity Center when Sylvester comes running in. Even here, among the quirky kids of Valley View, he looks like someone from another world, eyes wide and lit up, body in constant motion. We sit around the table—me, Roland, Darren, Kieran, Richard, Kirk, Annie and Sylvester sitting together. Kirk starts to go over interesting things that happened over the weekend. Darren got a used car, and he got a really good price on it. The only flaw is a minor problem with one of the engine mounts. Kieran, who is really into cars, launches into an explanation of how a mechanic would go about fixing the problem. It's hard to get him off this topic.

"Drop the car, Kieran," Kirk says after a while. "Drop the car."

At this point in Kieran's explanation, the hypothetical mechanic fixing the car is underneath the car. "If you're underneath it and you drop it," Kieran points out, "you DIE."

"You know," Kirk points out, "sometimes people with Asperger's get so in their own thoughts that they have a hard time listening to others. Sometimes you have to listen to other people talking—"

"What I was saying IS important," Kieran snarls.

"Not as important as keeping the school open. SHUT UP," Roland says, laying down the law. Kieran quiets.

We all know that for Valley View to stay open as a school, we need to be covering certain academic material. We shift to the subject of Current Events, going through the day's newspaper and talking about what's going on in politics.

"I want you to be patriotic," Kirk says. "Kieran does this. I see it. He goes to protests almost every week."

"What we really need to watch out for is Japan, pretty soon it will be all about Japan with their piece-of-shit rice cars—" Darren recognizes the shift in Kieran's voice as he starts to get worked up again and goes *shhhhhhh.*

By this time, Sylvester has put his head down in his arms. Annie looks at me, sadly. She murmurs to him about putting his head up, and he does. "Do you want to draw?" she asks him. He nods. She hands him a pad and a pencil, and he starts drawing as we shift to talking about global warming.

For all he can't quite keep up, Sylvester really enjoys being at Valley View. "Can I have a half-day?" he asks Kirk eagerly at lunch. I know that he means: *Can I stay here?* He is using words from an earlier conversation he overheard, where Kirk told Annie that if a full day is too much for him to handle, he might be able to come to the school for half-days.

Kieran overhears this. "Can *I* have a half-day?" he asks Kirk mockingly. He means that he'd like to go home.

But Sylvester's not fitting in in the younger classroom. He stayed there for a little while in the morning but then made his way back in with the older kids in the afternoon. He wants to be with them, and no one's stopping him. We're reading a novel about buried treasure, and Kirk is giving us some background, telling us a story about the actual historical island that the novel is based on. Suddenly, something I don't see flies through the air and hits Kieran.

"WHO THREW THAT?" Kieran whirls around, faces the table, and takes a step forward menacingly. Roland fesses up. "YOU piece of *SHIT!*" Kieran picks up a chair and swings it in the air. All heads are turned toward him, but everyone is pretty calm—except Darren, who stands up and takes a step toward Kieran.

"You throw things all the *time,*" he says. He looks almost tearful.

Kirk stays calm. "Leave the corrections to me," he suggests to the group. "There's something I've been trying to tell you. I think you'll think it is interesting. This island . . ." He continues telling us about the island, about what was actually buried there: spices and fabric and things that might not even be worth much money to anyone anymore. Kieran calms, sits. A moment later, as Kirk reads from the book, I see Roland quietly apologize to Kieran, and the two of them shake hands.

A few minutes later, Kieran gets up and leaves to get a drink of water. Without missing a beat or even really changing his tone of voice, Kirk says, "Now Kieran's had his little meltdown. He's had a hard week, you know. His parents finally broke up—thank goodness in a way . . . So don't antagonize him, OK?"

"We're not arguing anymore," Roland explains.

"These are all kids who couldn't go anywhere else," Kirk tells me wearily at the end of Sylvester's day at Valley View as we're wrapping things up. He wants to start up a new classroom for Sylvester and for some of the other new kids who are coming into the school. "We've just got to find the place where he will fit just right." Over the following weeks, Kirk kept telling me not to worry, that they were going to fix him up, real good. But this was easier said than done. Kirk shared Annie's concerns about the classroom that Sylvester had been placed in by the Brookfield district administrators. But he worried that Sylvester wouldn't fit in with the other kids at Valley View either.

Valley View had started out small but had grown as Kirk had taken on more and more tough cases. In the process, the composition of the school's population had also changed, broadening as the definition of "Asperger's syndrome" became more diffuse and more continuous with the rest of the "autism spectrum." The school had gone from being initially made up mostly of students like Darren, who met the prototypical Asperger's syndrome profile—academically gifted, socially awkward, logical-minded, and tending toward obsessiveness—to serving students who had a wider range of challenges: explosive tempers, learning difficulties. Some of the original students and their families had noticed this, and felt concerned about what had been lost. The balance between being inclusive and being specific was thus an ongoing tension.

You've Got to Look Out, La-La-La

Despite the growing diversity of the students in Asperger's classrooms, however, a few characteristics were shared by enough of the community members that it led to a distinctive classroom ethos—one that I remembered from the Journeyfolk Aspie Camp and went on to observe at some other autistic community spaces as well. These spaces were characterized by the tendency to remember and repeat certain discursive fragments, a pattern of attention that tends to stick on a single compelling stimulus for a long time, and the brittle, quick-to-snap affect that worsens over repeated and often mysterious experiences of social exclusion. A well-earned suspiciousness toward an unpredictable and often unwelcoming social world interacts with emotional volatility and a tendency toward mimetic repetition to create what I came to think of as a sort of echolalia chamber, resulting in the deep entrenchment of certain stances within autistic communities. In this case, youth within the community were socialized into an intense fear and distrust toward an educational system that they understood to be dangerous and adversarial.

By mid-October, Sylvester still wasn't in school. Annie and I took him on a lot of educational outings. She was still trying to homeschool him, but it was getting harder and harder on both of them. She attributed some of the trouble to his "tween stuff"—he was starting to shoot up like a beanstalk as puberty hit—and part to his depression and frustration at being out of school for so long.

"I guess he feels like he doesn't belong," she said to me. "Maybe even that nobody wants him—like an outcast." The Unity Center was officially closed down now, so he could no longer even do fun weekend events there with the Journeyfolk. Kirk still hadn't opened the new classroom at Valley View—according to Annie, he was struggling to find the funds to hire another teacher. Meanwhile, the attorney had started suggesting that Sylvester try the classroom that the district had proposed on the theory that if he tried it and failed spectacularly, it would bolster their case. "Now whenever the name [of that classroom] comes up, Sylvester says he feels like he's going to throw up. He's terrified of that time out room. He knows it's not appropriate, that there are no other autistic kids there—he wants to be with his peers! And he might be in physical danger because of other students picking on him because of his Asperger's."

But Sylvester wasn't feeling so good about Valley View either. "After that first day, they turned their backs on us," he told me as we walked through the local historic district, autumn leaves crunching under our feet. *Turned their backs on us* was an unusually abstract turn of phrase for Sylvester. I asked him what he meant. "They didn't do something they were supposed to do, so something happened. It's kind of a rip-off." In Sylvester's words—his fears of the time-out room, his metaphors of abandonment—I heard echoes of Annie's.

The process I observed in Brookfield, in which the kids' socialization into their diagnostic identities involved deep anxiety about being harmed by school, may be shared by a wide variety of youth who develop differently from what their culture considers to be the norm. But the characteristics of autism itself also contribute in particular ways to the amplification of discourses of betrayal and threat. This process involves not only the people diagnosed with autism spectrum conditions but also the wide spectrum of those who possess similar traits, who also come together around these kinds of environments. Valley View, for example, tended to attract people (this author, for one) who resonated with its quirky social ethos and felt an affinity with its intriguing, challenging students. Kirk himself identified as having Asperger's. ("The blind leading the deaf," Kieran commented caustically to me. "Write *that* in your book!") Who else among the volunteers teaching at the school might also be somewhere on the autism spectrum was a source of ongoing conjecture among the students.

The ecosystem of the Asperger's schools was also full of family members of the students. Some volunteered at the programs their kids attended, like Annie had done at the Unity Center. Most were in frequent communication with each other, sharing tips and tricks and advice and commiseration about the challenges they faced. Relatives of people on the spectrum, particularly first-degree relatives—parents, siblings—are significantly more likely to be on the autism spectrum themselves. Even those who never receive a diagnosis are more likely to display certain traits associated with autism at a milder level—a phenomenon called the "broader autism phenotype," or BAP for short (de Jonge et al., 2015; see also Constantino & Todd, 2003). While not all first-degree relatives of people diagnosed with autism spectrum conditions display BAP, some sizable proportion—most studies place the number at about 30% to 40%—show signs of autism in subclinical, often nonimpairing forms (Losh et al., 2017).

People who exhibit BAP are more likely to prefer solitary activities, to do poorly on tests requiring them to infer emotional states from facial expressions, and to have difficulty in social relationships. Some studies suggest that they are more likely to have a hard time shifting their attention from one thing to another and disengaging their attention from a stimulus once their attention has been captured by it. They also have a number of distinctive strengths—they tend to do well on tasks requiring close attention to visual detail and display unusually good memory for nonsocial stimuli—but these have been not been as thoroughly studied. Although it can bring benefits (many relatives of people on the autism spectrum pursue career fields where these attributes are valued), this style can cause problems in sociocultural settings that demand a high degree of social sensitivity, flexibility, and rapid shifts of attention. First-degree relatives of people with autism are significantly more likely to be diagnosed with a diverse range of psychiatric conditions, such as obsessive-compulsive disorder, anxiety, social phobia, and depression, even before the birth of the family member diagnosed with autism (see Sucksmith et al., 2011, for a review of these findings). When their personality traits are measured through standardized assessment instruments, they are significantly more likely than parents of children with other disabilities to appear anxious, impulsive, aloof, overly sensitive, irritable, and eccentric (Murphy et al., 2000).

This set of tendencies has implications for the social, emotional, and political life of autism communities. Concepts and phrases, fragments of discourse, and their implications get picked up and repeated, bounced back and forth, and amplified in a feedback loop that can get extremely loud. Corrective information is not always quickly recognized, opinions do not gently shift, and interpersonal comfort is not easily given and received. Miscommunications are frequent; intentions get misread. In some cases, uncertainty about the intentions and motivations of others encourages a socially transformative commitment to explicit, less-ambiguous communication among autistic communities; social anthropologist Ben Belek (2018) writes about a support group, run by and for people on the autism spectrum, where this took place. But in spaces where autistic people, sort-of-autistic people, and people who are not identified as autistic (who might not feel under any obligation to adjust their communication style) mix under fraught circumstances, a shared set of anxieties can heighten with remarkable speed and intensity.

A year after my initial fieldwork, I returned to Valley View for a follow-up visit. Many of the older students had graduated and moved on to entry-level jobs or community college, but they still kept in touch; the night before I arrived, Kirk told me, Kieran, Darren, and Roland had all been on a conference call about their plans to travel together to a car show. Stan had run out of money and had to go get a job where he could get paid; the school had been reduced to a single classroom, and Kirk was teaching it with help from a volunteering local politician. The day I arrived, we all worked on building a tower from the World's Fair for that year's project on the Seven Wonders of the World. As we painted, Kirk told me "a really terrible story" about a family who had twins, both on the autism spectrum. It was a cautionary tale: Both parents had died unexpectedly, within a short time, and they had no will and no legal documentation of the twins' diagnosis. So now the kids couldn't get services for their autism. "You never know what can happen," Kirk told me. "You've got to look out." Erin, a giggly 9-year-old who had recently joined the class, liked to take things people said and put them into song. "You've got to look out!" she sang back to him. "La-la-la-la!" I wondered how much she understood.

Lucy, however, understood a great deal about the system around her. Lucy's mother, Millie, was well known in Brookfield as a fierce and savvy advocate for her kids, both of whom were on the autism spectrum and attended Valley View. Millie often helped out at Valley View, and we heard a lot about the battles she was waging with the school district. During my visit, Lucy's class was reading George Orwell's (1945) *Animal Farm*. Lucy was really into *Animal Farm*. It had all her favorite elements: animals, conflictual relationships, injustice. As Kirk encouraged the students to think about the piece as an allegory for 20th-century politics, calling our attention to the connections between Snowball the pig and Leon Trotsky, Lucy was finding correlations closer to home. "This sounds like the school board!" she announced. "Let's chase Steve Marshall under the fence." Steve Marshall was a school board administrator, and she was suggesting he share Snowball's fate of being run out of town, never to be seen again.

For all their constant grumbling about the work, the kooky teachers, the chaos, and the weirdness of their classmates, the students at Valley View cherished the feeling of safety it provided them in a dangerous world. Gunnar, who had shot up about a foot in height and grown a massive mop of red hair since our days playing together at the Journeyfolk camp the previous year, had also joined the classroom by the time I came back to visit. He and Erin had a joking, play-fighting relationship that felt like it was always skating the edge of exploding into actual conflict. He poked her; she shrieked; he busted out of the room because he couldn't stand the noise of her shrieking. Everyone seemed to be keeping an eye on them. At one point, during a dodgeball game, there was a long, hold-your-breath moment when the two of them stood across from each other, her cringing and squeaking at him towering over her, holding a ball. Will one of them freak out? Will they have the courage to play with each other? He gently, gently, tapped her with the ball. She quietly, just above a whisper, screamed.

It was a lovely moment, and the kind of thing that could only happen in a place where kids have the time to get to know each other, to experiment, and to learn this kind of mutual self-regulation. Valley View was that kind of place: somewhere that students can explore themselves and their relationships with others and feel safe doing it. At one point, earlier in the game, Erin had let out a real shriek, and it looked like she was getting genuinely upset. "It's OK," Gunnar said to her, as always a little exasperated but also very gentle and very, very serious. "*No one will ever hurt you here.*"

Barely Special

"The other day, my mother said something hysterical to me," Greg said in a follow-up interview when I met up with him some years later. Now a young adult, he had gone to college and become a reasonably successful car salesman. He still lived at home with his parents, but a change was in the works, he told me: They wanted to move out of town for their retirement, and he wanted to stay in the community where he had grown up. So he and his parents were in the midst of the difficult process of figuring out if they could each live on their own. "She said, 'Greg, you're barely special.'" He laughed, riffing on the way the word *special* can be both a compliment and a euphemism. "What kind of mom would say to her kid: *You're barely special! You're not really special!*"

Greg's joke captures the multiplicity of Asperger's syndrome: the way it functions as both a stigmatized developmental disability and an identifier that evokes unusual ability as well as disorder. His joke also exemplifies the bricolage wit of Aspie culture, a community of disassembling and reassembling systems of discourse, of building and tinkering. In these spaces, broken things can be put back together. And kids who have come to think of themselves as broken can reassemble in a place where they are recognized and valued for a more complete, comprehensive picture of who they are—a version of autism that is not only about separation but also about attraction.

Sylvester wound up spending his sixth-grade year in what Annie described as a special education classroom at the local middle school. She thought it was OK—many of Sylvester's classmates had learning disabilities that were more pronounced than his, and she wished the teachers had more training in how to manage students' behaviors—but he wasn't having meltdowns like he had in his last school, and both of them were relieved that "the nightmare" of his time out of school was over. Sylvester himself was still wistful about the possibility of going to a school for kids on the autism spectrum. Later that year, I asked him how school was going and he said he hated it and he couldn't wait for it to be over.

"School's not going well, huh?"

"No," he replied very seriously, "they don't have autism training."

"Hm!" I said. "What kind of autism training should they have?" He shrugged. "What do you wish they knew about autism?" He shrugged again. "What would be different about a school where there was autism training?"

"The other kids would be autistic."

"And how would that be different?"

"More fun."

Sylvester had learned that autistic spaces were places where he could be with others like him who share common interests and feel accepted. Autism-specific programs offered Sylvester and his peers a little protection from the constant, corrosive movement from classroom to classroom and from the threats to safety and identity posed by placement in a community defined only by support needs that are equated with failure. These programs offered these kids a fuller picture of who they are, characterized by strengths as well as vulnerabilities—and, at the same time, maintained a clear contrasting narrative about who they are *not*. This manifestation of autistic community suggested to Sylvester and his peers the possibility that there was, after all, somewhere they belonged.

3

Innocent Machines

It's a Brain Developmental Thing, You Know What I Mean?

It's a busy day at ASPEN.[1] Emily the assistant teacher and I have grabbed a rare quiet moment to talk while the students are at lunch. We sit among the wild art projects the students have cooked up, surrounded by collages of Easter Bunny–ninja–robot–clowns and big cushy bean-bag chairs, in the little nook set aside for students to take a breather if they start to get stressed out or overwhelmed. As we begin our interview, I ask her: *"How would you define Asperger's syndrome?"*

Emily is not sure how to answer, struggling to put her practical wisdom into words. She has only been working with this population for a few years and considers herself anything but an expert, although her combination of warm camaraderie and limit-setting straight talk gets her a good bit of respect from her students. A breakthrough comes, however, when I ask her about her prior work history. She draws a comparison that I heard frequently around her school district: between the students in ASPEN, all of whom have been diagnosed with Asperger's syndrome or a similar autism spectrum condition, and the other group of students with whom they share a building: the students in the "Pathways" program. These students are classified as "psychiatrically identified," and their education program is administered collaboratively with a local psychiatric hospital for children and adolescents. In the eyes of Emily and many of the other teachers and families involved in the ASPEN program, the Pathways students were everything the Asperger's students were not.

> EMILY: Alice [the other teacher] and I were upstairs on the third
> floor with Pathways, which is emotionally—well, I don't want to say
> *disturbed*, but—I forget what the term is, these days—emotionally
> fragile, kids that were under the supervision of Marden Psychiatric

Clinic. And they, you know, they had a social worker—of course [the Asperger's students] do, too, but—they would go out and see a psychiatrist, you know, a lot of them were on medication. Which some of them here are, too—so it was just like, more of: the way they were was probably a product of their home life, how they were brought up, what they'd been put through, maybe some chemically—you know, they mighta had hyper-whatever.

[The Pathways students] were more difficult than these guys. They were all work-avoidants. These [Asperger's] guys, most of them *like* to do the work. And they like to get it done. They don't seem to smoke, or—you know, the other kids in Pathways, they're always running out for cigarettes. . . . It's nice! It's a nice change. I enjoy them, actually.

As Emily works to articulate the difference between these two groups, she tries to put a commonsense understanding into words, frequently referencing the shared nature of this understanding: *They see a psychiatrist, you know?* But both groups see psychiatrists and social workers. Both take medication. The shared understanding of what truly differentiates them—the schema that Emily is attempting to bring from implicit to explicit—is about more than what they do; it's about why they are the way they are.

What really matters, as she goes on to explain, is this: The problems of the Pathways kids, and their solutions, arise out of fluid, shifting, malleable things, such as their life experiences and their brain chemicals. The Asperger's difference, on the other hand, is hardwired into the material structure of the brain, fixed and impervious to the vicissitudes of pharmacological and interpersonal chemistry. This distinction turns out to have wide-ranging implications for how the behavior of each set of students is interpreted and treated.

ELIZABETH: What do you think accounts for those differences, between the Asperger's kids and the Pathways kids?
EMILY: Now the Asperger's—well, that's a whole *brain* developmental thing, isn't it. So that alone, I believe, would alter their behavior. And that's just the way they're gonna be. You know what I mean? I think the Pathways kids—theirs is a *learned* behavior. You know? Where they *learned* to be work avoidant. Or they've been told: "You're noth-

ing but a piece of crap," all their lives, so they act out that way. These guys [gesturing to the ASPEN classroom], I think they will *always* have that. The way they act. As they get older, they can compensate for it a bit. But the other ones, at Pathways, they should be able to— they *could* learn to do the right thing. Depending on if they get out of their environment at home. They have fine families, the Asperger's [students], and it's not because of—but then again, their behaviors aren't bad! They're just different, you know, they're just different. And who's really to say who's normal, and who's different. We're all different, you know? And that's fine, it makes it more interesting. . . . I think it's more of: this is who they are. And that's not really going to change. Unless—I mean, there's not a medication, to fix Asperger's— and they don't *want* to be fixed! You know? I mean, I don't think [they do]. That's who they are and they *like* who they are.

Emily's description of the differences between the students in her Asperger's classroom and the students in the Pathways program exemplifies a powerful and pervasive discourse, both within and outside her school district, about the differences between people diagnosed with developmental disabilities and people diagnosed with psychiatric disorders. Her description tells us a great deal not only about the attributes that she observes among particular groups of students but also about the presumed relationships between these attributes.

The etiological status of Asperger's syndrome as a "brain developmental thing" leads Emily directly to her conclusion that "that's just the way they're gonna be. You know what I mean?" What she means—and the conclusion that she assumes I will draw as well—is twofold. First, the characteristics and dispositions specific to the Asperger's students are rooted in their brain development, more so than would be the case for other groups. Second, the solid and robust physicality of this brain difference, its imperviousness to outside forces such as medication, motivates a stance of accepting the students—"Who's to say who's normal?"—rather than futile attempts at changing them. Because the differences exhibited by the Asperger's students arise out of the physical makeup of the brains they were born with, their differences aren't considered bad; they are "just different." But while these differences may exist outside a moral evaluative system of good or bad, right or wrong, they are nonetheless viewed favorably, as both enjoyable and productive. These students like to do the work and like to get it done instead of always running out for cigarettes; it's nice.

The Pathways students, on the other hand, do not only behave differently; they exist within an entirely different ontological and interpretive paradigm. Their problems are understood as learned behavior, rooted in family conflict, which manifests "chemically" and responds to psychiatric treatment. Their way of being is perceived as fluid, malleable, and open to outside influence. Along with their capacity for change, responsiveness, and intersubjectivity comes culpability. Emily's evaluation of their behaviors arises not out of relativist tolerance but out of a sense that there is a "right thing" and the belief that they can, and should, learn to do it. They are moral, intentional agents, shaped by the social world and therefore responsible for their participation within it.

Both the "Pathways kids" and the students in the Asperger's classroom are strongly identified with the classifications that have been placed on them. These classifications determine their educational trajectories, as well as a great deal of their daily context: who will be their classmates, how they will be taught, what opportunities will be presented to them. Both sets of classifications draw on ideas about how, and why, we become who we are. These ideas have been heavily shaped by disciplines that study the mind: psychology, educational sciences, psychiatry, neuroscience. But the tradition that each classification draws on is different. The "brain development things" of the ASPEN students are considered to be developmental disabilities; the Pathways kids are considered to have mental health disorders. These two domains are associated with different funding streams, different treatment infrastructures, different metaphorical entailments, and different moral valences. The students living under these descriptions not only occupy two different classrooms; they also occupy two different *brainhoods*.

Who Are the People in Your Brainhood?

I have taken the term *brainhood* from Fernando Vidal (2009), who describes "the ascendancy, throughout industrialized and highly medicalized societies, of a certain view of the human being . . . specified by the property of 'brainhood,' i.e. the property or quality of *being*, rather than simply *having*, a brain" (p. 6). Along with Francisco Ortega (Ortega & Vidal, 2007, 2011; Vidal & Ortega, 2017), he posits a "cerebral subject" whose self-identification is deeply shaped by both the "psy-"disciplines (psychology, psychiatry) and the network of practices within which they are embroiled. Throughout this book, I have pluralized the term to emphasize the extent to which different diagnoses are situated in different intellectual traditions of knowledge production, leading to different conceptualizations of the relationship between brain and behavior. Thus, individuals living under the description of these differing diagnoses are enrolled in and inhabit differing "brainhoods."

When I use the term *brainhood* in this sense, I refer to a cluster of interrelated representations of the brain as a symbol of the self. Brainhoods are situated within some particular intellectual history and tradition (i.e., psychoanalysis, neuroscience, behaviorism, etc.) or potentially at their points of intersection. They are organized around a metaphorical schema that suggests a particular kind of robust physicality (the brain as a series of wires, as a chemical soup, as a container for a deep and unknown unconscious, etc.). They motivate particular responses (accommodation, chemical modulation, insight-oriented psychotherapy, etc.), and these responses are situated within (and, at times, across or between) particular resource infrastructures (an Office of Developmental Disabilities, an affluent or under-resourced school system, a private psychotherapy practice that accepts certain insurances, etc.). All brainhoods exist in relation to other brainhoods—perhaps overlapping with them, perhaps existing on the other side of town from them, or perhaps looming on the wrong side of the tracks.

In a critique of Vidal's (2009) concept of "brainhood," Nikolas Rose and Joelle Abi-Rached (2013) have suggested that the contemporary imperative is not so much that we *be* our brains but that we *have* our brains—and that we take the responsibility to care for and work on them in various ways. Brainhoods, on the other hand, as I am using the term here, are not so much something we *have* as much as something we *inhabit*. Suggesting that one *has* a neurochemical brain emphasizes the aspects of its parameters that slosh around within the interior of one's own body; what follows is instead a story about people who *occupy* particular territories that are set up and delineated in particular ways. Like neighborhoods, brainhoods are multiple. Their boundaries overlap and are frequently contested. That being said, any given person is unlikely to be hanging out in too many of them at the same time.

The single building that holds both the ASPEN students and the Pathways students also holds multiple brainhoods, which the students learn to occupy. In the classrooms at Brookfield, where students are classified according to how their brains are presumed to work, kids learn that *how they learn* is a big part of what makes them *who they are*. And one of the things they learn is that it matters very much whether they are classified as having a *mental illness* or a *developmental disability*. In Brookfield and beyond, this distinction comes with powerful connotations: Developmental disabilities, unlike mental illnesses, are innate, faultless, and fixed.

We Knew It Wasn't Your Fault for Being Mentally Retarded

The concept of developmental disability is a fairly recent one. It emerged during the second half of the 20th century, as state services for what was then called "mental hygiene" and services for what was then called "mental retardation" became increasingly separate entities, culminating in the 1970s with the formation of two separate state offices to administer these services (see Castellani, 2005, for an in-depth history of this process). These two agencies had somewhat similar roles and mandates, but they offered different services and operated under a different set of assumptions. The office serving people with mental retardation gradually expanded to other lifelong, early-onset conditions such as cerebral palsy, for the most part remaining geared toward serving those who would need significant support throughout the rest of their lives.

Martina Grace, a psychologist in a nearby city whose career focuses on working with people with Asperger's, described it to me this way (her tone, in case it is not clear here, was one of wry critique):

> The reason that they [split the agencies, in the middle of the 20th century] is because we still thought that it was your fault for being mentally ill, and we knew it wasn't your fault for being mentally retarded. That's really how it came. And we also thought, "Well, if you're mentally retarded then it's forever. We're going to have to take care of you forever. We might as well get a plan set in motion to take care of you forever."

And mental illness, you hope people will get better, and you may not have to take care of them forever. So they had different—so the agencies split apart.

As the definition of developmental disability has broadened, however, these assumptions have become harder to sustain. In the last decades of the 20th century, the concept of "neurodevelopmental disability" began to expand the purview of this term into more subtle manifestations of difference, such as the "minimal brain dysfunctions" that would go on to be called attention-deficit/hyperactivity disorder, or ADHD (Lakoff, 2000) as well as specific learning disabilities and social cognitive disabilities such as Asperger's syndrome. This process complicated the mandate and mission of these agencies. Dr. Grace went on to say:

> Now of course, most of these agencies in most states are not just called *mental retardation*, they're called something about *developmental disabilities*. And so all these things that are *developmental disabilities*, they also theoretically need to address. But it's become more difficult as we think of other things like learning disabilities, and ADHD, and all these other things. Well, are those developmental disabilities? Do we need to take care of people like that? Well, yeah, you need to take care of somebody who's ADHD who can't take care of themselves, but the vast majority of people with ADHD are doing just fine. Well, that's the same with Asperger's syndrome. Lots of people are doing just fine—and the ones who aren't, need support.

Splitting the agencies has made it difficult for those who do not fall neatly into one category or the other. "Now they're realizing that was probably a mistake in some ways," Dr. Grace said. "It made people fall through the cracks who had both."

In some ways, autism spectrum conditions occupy a contested middle ground between mental health disorder and developmental disability. This is especially true for conditions of the Asperger's sort, as the challenges faced and posed by people with such diagnoses often involve dramatic dysregulations of moods, behaviors, and relationships rather than (or in addition to) more global functional impairments. And autism, of course, has a particularly troubled history with the question of blame. Autism was for a time attributed to parenting failures, and the renunciation of this perspective has been so thorough that it has produced a particular emphasis on the ways in which autism is innate, inborn, and neurogenetically determined. In a system within which developmental disabilities are understood as both faultless and permanent, and mental health concerns are fluid and morally valenced with complex questions of culpability and agency, autism spectrum conditions are often placed firmly in the former category.

The Little Professors

As "brain developmental things," autism spectrum conditions also evoke a particular set of lay conceptions of neuroscience, particularly notions of the brain as a fixed physiological system whose hidden workings are gradually being discovered through cutting-edge visualization technologies and consistently replicable scientific experimentation. They evoke what Tobias Rees (2010) refers to as the "*regime fixiste*": the vision, dominant throughout the 20th century, of the brain as "a fixed and immutable machine" (p. 156). As people with Asperger's syndrome live under such technoscientific descriptions, they also perform and exemplify them, in a heightened form of what Hacking (1995) would call "the looping effect of human kinds."

The association between Asperger's syndrome and a particular way of doing science—an approach to the world characterized by repetition, systematic classification, a de-emphasis of subjectivity and contextual embedding, and a selective attention to fixed systems—is long-standing, beginning with the very birth of the category. Asperger's syndrome was named after pediatrician Hans Asperger, who, in 1944, identified a "highly recognizable type of child" whom he nicknamed "the little professors" due to their combination of obsessive, circumscribed interests, social clumsiness, and pedantic speech. He noted that many of these children were also capable of "unswerving determination and penetrating intellectual powers" which could lead to "outstanding achievements in their chosen areas" such as astronomy and mathematics (Asperger, 1947/1991, p. 88). Similarly, along with his colleagues, Simon Baron-Cohen, one of the first psychological researchers to write extensively about Asperger's syndrome, (Baron-Cohen, Richler, Bisarya, Gurunathan, & Wheelwright, 2003) has characterized it as a tendency toward systematizing—an effective way of analyzing the "law-governed inanimate universe" of predictable inputs and outputs—over empathizing, defined as "the drive to identify another person's emotions and thoughts, and to respond to those with an appropriate emotion" (p. 361). He and his colleagues note that a tendency toward systemizing can, in some individuals, lead to impressive achievements in "factual, scientific, technical, or rule-based subjects" (Baron-Cohen et al., 2003, p. 363).

Conceptualizations of Asperger's syndrome as both hardwired in the brain and characterized by an attention to the structured, predictable aspects of objectively knowable realities over messy subjectivities also resonate with entrenched epistemological stances within the psy-disciplines. In particular, the idea of people with Asperger's as scientific in a way that privileges predictability over subjectivity evokes contemporary depictions of neuroscience—and, to a somewhat lesser extent, genetics—as offering an opportunity to ground our knowledge of human variation in an objective and replicable science of the physical body (e.g., see Cuthbert, 2014; Insel & Quirion, 2005). In his ethnographic study of early brain visualization technologies, anthropologist of science Joseph Dumit (2004) observes how much of the appeal of these technologies rests on the "taboo nature of subjectivity in science" in which "every possibility of subjectivity must be eliminated in order to produce something reliable—that is, something real, something known" and a subsequent romanticizing of "automation, which stands as the opposite of interactivity" (p. 122). Locating the self and its vicissitudes within a body whose physical properties are governed by predictable laws allows for not only reliability but also protection from moral judgment. In her ethnographic study of the training of psychiatry residents caught between psychodynamic and biological paradigms, anthropologist Tanya Luhrmann (2000) notes that these different paradigms evoke deep-rooted and pervasive ideas about bodies and minds. She summarizes these ideas as follows: "If something is in the body the individual cannot be blamed; the body is always morally innocent. If something is in the mind, however, it can be controlled and mastered, and a person who fails to do so is morally at fault" (p. 8).

Within the two groups of students in the ACER building (ACER is the acronym for Brookfield's special education services), the ontological assumptions and traditions of knowledge production underlying each group's diagnosis organize the interpretations of each group's behaviors into a neat and compelling parallel. Brains, as understood by a psychiatric science driven by replicable experimentation on fixed physical systems, are material, predictable, and morally innocent—just like the Asperger's students that best enact and exemplify them. The minds and behaviors of the "psychiatric" kids, on the other hand, are seen as unpredictable, fluid, socially embedded, morally culpable, and messily human—reflecting the psychiatric traditions out of which their classifications developed.

The Value to Society of Someone Who Is Very Logical

The Asperger's students' enactment and exemplification of a value-producing technoscience did a great deal of rhetorical work throughout the Brookfield school system. It marshaled and protected scarce resources for the students diagnosed with Asperger's. It helped establish a designated space where these students could find community and acceptance. It also helped make sense of their often-perplexing behaviors, softening the impact of the interpersonal conflicts that often followed and surrounded them. And it helped conjure a vision of their future employment prospects. Commentary on what made the Asperger's students distinctive often involved spontaneous interpretations of the labor market, its changing nature, and its centrality to the students' futures.

Annabelle is an administrator within the ACER system. Her job is to place students who have special needs into academic and vocational programs and to make sure they get the supports they need there. In my interview with her, she observed an affinity between students with Asperger's and technology so intense and intimate as to be almost symbiotic:

> I've seen students come through the building with Asperger's who've excelled in computer design classes, exceeded expectations, and then gone on to college successfully, in a computer field as well. And I have a few kids integrated into classrooms, I have one who's actually fairly severely autistic, who's excelling amazingly in the computer area, whose teachers

actually think would be highly employable in a repair and networking job. And I had another student who was extremely successful in the computer repair class. And so it is seeming to me that the trend is definitely technological at this point, in computers.

And I just find that interesting because I wonder what that means, really. I'm wondering: is society, is humankind even more so needing people who have Asperger's syndrome? And somehow is this biologically driven as an evolutionary thing? . . . Because [Asperger's] is on the rise so much that you can almost see the value to society of someone who's very logical and not as emotional. I think that in the techie society, it may be a fitting adaptation in some ways.

What is striking about Annabelle's hypothesis is not only her observation, shared among many within Brookfield and outside it, that Asperger's students seem to gravitate toward technology and work effectively and well with it. She also proposes that there is some fundamental *simpatico* between people with Asperger's and this technology, imagining that they are in some way made to go with computers, born into a biologically determined symbiosis of human and technology. In this way, they provide "value to society" and may even, surprisingly, be "highly employable."

This understanding about Asperger's, technology, and value takes on a self-fulfilling power as it guides Annabelle in her job duties: allocating the scarce resources available to Brookfield special education services according to student needs. Brookfield is not a particularly affluent school district, and the sense among students in special education, especially, was that they frequently got the short end of the stick. Students routinely used the word *ACER* as a joking term for things that were broken, busted, past their prime: An "ACER pen" would be one with no ink left in it; an "ACER computer" is one that runs slowly, has an outdated operating system, and/or is full of viruses. The phrase, as the students used it, referred obliquely not only to themselves—as broken, as less useful, as not quite right, as disposable—but also to the fact that a lot of the materials within ACER really weren't well maintained or up-to-date. This was not the case, however, within ASPEN, whose staff were justifiably proud of their access to cutting-edge tools and technology. Program administrators and parents often told me about situations in which a student with a particular vocational interest related to technology—game design, architecture—was able to get access through ASPEN to high-quality new software or other tools related to that interest. The student–teacher ratio in the ASPEN classrooms was quite low, enabling students to work through material at their own pace and teachers to customize lessons to students' particular interests. The discourse of Asperger's students as young technologists in the making moved significant resources in their direction.

One of the resources afforded the ASPEN program was the opportunity for staff to attend training on how to better understand and teach students on the autism spectrum; this was an advantage frequently cited by parents who wanted their kids to go there. Early on in my time at ASPEN, I attended one such training, held by a local ad hoc committee of autism professionals working to raise awareness and educate the Brookfield community (I had been sitting in on their monthly meetings while I was in Brookfield). This particular event featured a videotaped presentation by Tony Attwood, a dryly funny Australian clinician who was one of the first to bring Asperger's syndrome to widespread attention. Insightful, clinically astute, and displaying a refreshing sense of empathy and appreciation for these frequently misunderstood kids, Attwood and his witty and vivid lectures contributed to establishing the prototypical clinical picture of the Aspie kid as mechanistic and innocent, a computer with a particular processing style.

"Computers," the cheerful gentleman in the video told us, "were designed by and for people with Asperger's syndrome. Why? Because you don't have to socialize with it. It does not get moody. Unlike teachers, it does not get premenstrual tension, or hangovers . . . . The major way of learning is visual and logical. Not emotional. Emotion and logic are contradictory. . . . Computer science may be a very appropriate career choice for many of these individuals who find the logic of computers is just so natural to them" (Attwood, 2002). This association of Asperger's students with logical technology over emotion-laden sociality resonated throughout the Brookfield district, with tangible consequences for the students.

The discourse of Asperger's students as computing machines estranged from sociality also served as an explanatory model that offered a rationale for their frequent social blunders, differentiating their innocent mistakes from the knowing transgressions of the morally culpable.

"A lot of such children's behavior appears rude, inconsiderate, lawless, naughty, Badly Brought Up—but they're just not aware how their behavior affects other people," Attwood (2002) explains in the training video. He then shares a vignette, which I quote at length because it has become somewhat famous in the clinical lore of Asperger's:

> Quite often the child doesn't understand the codes of conduct, those unwritten rules that tell you you talk to your teacher in one way, your school principal another way, and the other children—and they approach everybody the same way. And they don't seem to understand—and I'll give you an illustration we had with a child who was with his mother at a supermarket checkout. And in this situation, he spotted a lady, in front of him and pointed to her, and in a very loud voice, heard throughout the supermarket, said: "Isn't she fat!!!" His mother then said "Sh! sh! you don't say that!" To which he replied in an equally loud voice: "But she IS fat!" [This droll recounting got a good laugh from the audience]. Now: several things occurred here. First of all, he was not aware of how that comment would affect the feelings of the person in question. It was not malicious, it was not nasty, he was just stating the obvious: *isn't she fat?* Secondly his mother's signals of *ssh ssh—you don't say that—I'm embarrassed* were equally not picked up. And finally, the child was perplexed that he was being chastised for telling the truth. She *is* fat! And these children are self-appointed revealers of the truth. They tell you exactly everything.

Of course, the child in this vignette did *not* tell exactly everything. He did not point out that the gum packet was green, or that people were standing in line, or that the food cost money. The child instead chose to focus on a stimulus that he knew to be remarkable: a woman's body that deviated from expected norms. This vignette is being held up as an example of a child who treats everyone in exactly the same way, regardless of social role; it is actually a story about drawing a very specific social distinction. However, depicting the child as a transparent input–output machine erases many of the significances of his utterance.

This occlusion of social meaning within Asperger's faux pas frequently supports the differentiation of developmental disability from the misbehavior of those with mental illness. Attwood (2002), in the training video, goes out of his way to draw this distinction when recommending occasional long weekends and additional school holidays for Asperger's kids who are overwhelmed by the demands of socializing in school. "For some," he says, "the degree of stress is enormous, and they need what I call mental health breaks. That's not to say they're mentally ill. These kids are different. They are not mad, bad, or defective. *They are just different*." Value-neutral Aspie difference is explicitly contrasted here with a madness that is equated with badness and defectiveness; in the process, the morally meaningful resonances of Aspie communication is obscured. The mad and the bad are banished to their own categorical realm, contributing to the stigma they face as flawed moral agents. This distinction can be leveraged strategically, as it is here, in order to protect a precious resource: the opportunity for students on the autism spectrum to have some space of their own. In Brookfield, the fight for such a space often became deeply contentious.

They Act Out Because They're Stressed

Millie was one of several Brookfield parents in a prolonged court battle with the school district. Feisty and funny, she was fiercely protective of her two teenagers, Richard and Lucy, both of whom had been diagnosed with high-functioning autism spectrum disorders. Both children currently attended Valley View, where Millie also volunteered, and were very happy there; the district was trying to place Lucy at ASPEN. To get the school district to place Lucy at Valley View instead (thus covering the cost of tuition, which Millie would not have been able to pay out of pocket), Millie needed to demonstrate that there were no appropriate options for Lucy within the public school system. She was arguing this point in as many ways as she could; at one point, she picketed the district offices with a sign saying that they had violated her child's civil rights.

A great deal of the work that she did was rhetorical, building up and highlighting the perceived differences between her children on the autism spectrum and the children in the ACER system, particularly those who were classified as "ED," short for "emotional disturbance." While she had many concerns about the restrictiveness of the ACER building—the security guards, the locked bathrooms that kids needed permission to visit—she was most worried about proximity to the Pathways students, given the potential contagion of their misbehavior and the stigma of their moral responsibility.

> MILLIE: We're not placing her into ACER. You can basically forget it. There are a lot of children in these programs that are really inappropriate for these kids to be with, because [kids on the autism spectrum] are basically socially naive kids. They mirror other kids' actions. [Many of the available classroom placements] have autism and ED. And a lot of kids that have autism, are not ED.
>
> ELIZABETH: How do you see the difference between autism and emotional disturbance?
>
> MILLIE: I think a lot of these [autism spectrum] kids do act out, and they're classified as emotionally disturbed, because people don't know how to handle them. I think they act out because they're stressed. . . . A lot of these kids have the expressive language issues and they can't say: *This noise is just so much and I can't deal with the noise.* Or *These lights, it's just so much and I can't deal with these fluorescent lights, I can't deal with the buzzing, I can hear the humming of these lights.* And it's too much, it's too overwhelming, it's the sensory, is way too much. And people don't understand that the sensory overload is so much for them that they can't deal with it.
>
> ELIZABETH: And how do people interpret that?
>
> MILLIE: They interpret that he's acting out. People misinterpret it, basically. They think it's ED! They think it's, you know, just bad behavior. And of course, it's the mother's fault. Or it's the father's fault. It's family situations. You know. And that's what they try—blaming me—with Lucy.

The thing is, many of the students being considered for ASPEN *do* misbehave frequently, flying into extraordinary tantrums or stubbornly refusing to comply with teacher's requests—if they didn't, they could stay in a mainstream classroom and wouldn't be eligible for ACER in the first place. Accordingly, Millie must somehow make sense of their (emotional, rule-challenging) behavior in a way that preserves her sense of them as innocent and rule-bound, differentiating the meaning of their misbehavior from that of the "ED kids." She does so by using a metaphorical language of physical systems to describe the "acting out" of Asperger's students. They do not exhibit "bad behavior" but act out instead because they are "stressed," and stress leads to breakage. The environment they are stressed by is sensory, not interpersonal: fluorescent light, for example, or buzzing or noise. ED kids, on the other hand, inhabit a morally valenced world of emotional intersubjectivity; they act out because of "bad behavior." And such behavior, she notes, is prone to being interpreted as the fault of the parents. Interpreting Lucy's "acting out" as motivated by interpersonal factors rather than as a reaction to pure sensory input, therefore, has significant negative consequences, implicating and pathologizing not only Lucy but her entire family system as well.

Furthermore, it puts Lucy herself at risk for harm, if such interpretations should lead to her being placed in a classroom full of interpersonally violent students. Seeking refuge from bullying and other student-on-student violence was a reason that parents frequently cited for trying to get their kids into Asperger's-specific classrooms and out of classrooms for students with emotional or behavioral disturbances. At ASPEN and Valley View, the fact that many of the students had a history of being bullied by students with these classifications contributed to an overall sense of the Asperger's students as innocent victims and ED students as dangerous aggressors.

But not only is Lucy's physical and emotional well-being at risk if she is placed with these students; her behavioral repertoire may also be affected. The concern Millie voices, that Lucy will "mirror" the behaviors of these students if she is forced to spend too much time around them, was one I heard frequently in Asperger's-specific programs such as Valley View. The fear is that students with Asperger's who are placed in classrooms with ED students may start defying rules rather than compliantly following them; however, they will do so out of rote imitation of others rather than out of their own individual volition, perhaps even unaware of the meaning of their actions to others. If an ED student swears, they are doing so out of genuine hurt and anger; if an Asperger's student swears, they probably don't even know what the word means.

> MILLIE: You got a kid with high-functioning autism put into a program where they shouldn't be, and they do the wrong thing because they come up to someone and look them right in their face, and the

kid shoves them away and they get slammed—well, they don't know
the social cues! They don't know any better. . . . And they get put into
a program where you get some people that are—a little more street-
savvy . . . and they get their face beaten in every day. Of *course* you're
going to have nervous breakdowns and stuff.

Construing Lucy as innocent of social mores—as "not knowing any
better"—depicts her as a fundamentally different sort of sociomoral
entity from those who act out of their "street-savvy," their corrupt and
corrupting knowledge of the social world. Lucy's misbehavior is instead
interpreted as a reaction to the physical world, deterministically pre-
ordained by the sum total of the quantity of input she is getting minus
her system's capacity to cope. Her nervous breakdowns are an inevitable
consequence of ongoing strain.

Like many cultural schemas with profound personal and political
ramifications, the representation of people with Asperger's syndrome as
mechanistic, self-contained systems—as innocent machines—is both an
exaggeration and simplification of what its proponents overall know to be
true. Lucy enthusiastically asserts her own agency in social situations on
a regular basis, and Millie knows it, laughing with me about her determination, her creative storytelling, and her capacity to be "a total monster"
to her older brother when she isn't getting what she needs. As psychological anthropologist Claudia Strauss (2005) has observed, most people tend
to internalize and draw on multiple social discourses in their reasoning about complex situations, including those that seem to conflict with
each other on some points once they are each made explicit. The model
of Asperger's kids as innocent machines is only one thread in the complex tapestry of relationships connecting the Brookfield students to those
around them. However, it is a bright thread that runs through and unites
a number of contexts and conversations. It does a tremendous amount
of work: helping Millie send her children to a private school in a well-off
community and keep them away from the "street-savvy" public school-
ers of her socioeconomically depressed neighborhood, protecting spaces
where close relationships can be developed and nurtured over time, and
giving bright students who struggle academically a special relationship
with the power and prestige of technoscience. As such, it serves as a defense against multiple forms of social and economic precarity.

If You're Not Capable, You Can't Do It. So.

However, this conception of Asperger's students as innocent machines can also be deeply alienating. Majia Nadesan (2005), a scholar of communications and biopolitical governance who is herself the parent of a person on the autism spectrum, cautions us that imagining people on the autism spectrum as being fundamentally machinelike also connotes an estrangement from the interpretive, volitional, and social aspects of human life:

> The irremediable gap between actual computers and human brains typically situates in the fundamentally human capacities of sociality (love, desire, sympathy, empathy) and spontaneous imagination (play, aspirations, fantasy), and in reflexive "self-consciousness" (whose nature remains ambiguous). . . . Consequently, the semiotic equations across autism, technology/science, social deficiencies, and lack of personal reflexivity contain the potential to dehumanize autism and the people associated with this label. (p. 131)

The question of whether people with brain problems can be held responsible for their actions was much on the mind of Fred Kalinkas, stepfather of Allen, the sulky skateboarder at Valley View, when I interviewed him for this research study. Allen's diagnosis served as a powerful explanatory narrative in his family, transforming his mother's and stepfather's interpretations of him and his actions.

> FRED: I was skeptical [of the Asperger's diagnosis], at first. And thought it was always—behavioral problems. That was the first reaction. *He's just being a bad kid.* You know, so discipline is what's needed . . . I think that's part of the problem with behavioral kids is that parents don't recognize or don't have the resources to take an interest, so they become behavioral problems. . . . It took a while to diagnose him. They weren't sure what it was. And everyone else was trying to blame it on a behavioral problem.
>
> ELIZABETH: They were trying to blame it on a behavioral problem?
>
> FRED: Yeah. It's a behavioral problem not a—you know, he just was an uncooperative child! Even Corrine's [Allen's mother's] parents.

Even her aunt. You know, they still don't really believe that he has the Asperger's. They really don't see the real—most of the time.

The proper attribution of responsibility for Allen's outbursts requires differentiating the manifestations of Asperger's from the blameworthy behavior of a "bad kid" whose problem is caused by lack of discipline on the part of parents, operating in tandem with an intentional lack of cooperation on the part of the child. In Fred's view, Allen's relatives do not see "the real": that his defiance of social norms originates in the hidden setup of his neural mechanics, mechanics that we cannot see but only infer:

> FRED: The mind just doesn't work the way it's supposed to. It's a disconnect.
> ELIZABETH: A disconnect between . . . ?
> FRED: Between the receptors I suppose—It's not firing the way it's supposed to, right brain to left brain—whatever reason, you know, I don't know what the brain waves do. I think it's just that it doesn't quite connect the way it normally does.

Fred understands Allen's misbehaviors to be determined by mysterious failures of his brain rather than volitional, comprehensible, communicative gestures. Thus, he sees his stepson's behavior as determined by urges he cannot control and Allen himself as incapable of stopping his reactions:

> FRED: I think they're uncontrollable urges. Uncontrollable thoughts. They can't stop themselves. They say what they think. *We* learn to filter that stuff. Not say those things. *They* don't.
> ELIZABETH: Whereas a kid who had a behavioral problem but didn't have Asperger's—
> FRED: It's hard to say. Generally, it's a parental problem, I think. When the kid's capable but not asked to do the things he should be doing. But if you're not capable, you can't do it. So.

The moral absolution that accompanies Fred's interpretation of Allen's behavior as a biophysiological system driven by internal cause-and-effect logic rather than interpersonal participation brings deeply alienating consequences: He describes Allen as incapable of change, of self-control and thus belonging to a "they" fundamentally different from the capable, agentic "we" to which he and I belong. In such moments, the potential for change, for the capability to "do the things he should be doing," is foreclosed.

In *Recovery's Edge: An Ethnography of Mental Health Care and Moral Agency*, psychiatric anthropologist Neely Myers (2015) argues that a key component of mental health is *moral agency*: "the ability to be recognized as a 'good' person in a way that makes possible intimate connections to others" (p. 13). Only through relationships of mutual accountability, she argues convincingly, can we take our place as members of a community and thus live full lives. When students with Asperger's are conceptualized as fundamentally estranged from such networks of accountability, the meaningfulness of their communications becomes obscured. Under such circumstances, they are at risk for being reduced to what Marrow and Luhrmann (2012) have described as "bare voice": a form of "social marginalization [that] takes place by stripping away the subject's efficacy in social communication" (p. 493). They chronicle this "loss of communicative agency—the revocation of the privilege of being recognized as speaking meaning" (p. 511)—among women with psychosis in Chicago who are abandoned to the streets and people with psychosis in India who are abandoned within their own households: people in far less privileged circumstances than the Asperger's students. Yet the same system that rewarded, recognized, and amplified certain aspects of the Asperger's students' communications (those related to technology and compliance with rules) also simultaneously dismissed the significance of other aspects (those that posed social and interpersonal challenges), emptying them of social meaning.

These daily negotiations have moral, ethical, and political stakes that transcend the classroom. Several years ago, I attended a talk by the child psychologist Ross Greene, author of the very popular book *The Explosive Child* (1998) and developer of a model of "collaborative problem-solving" between adults and "behaviorally challenging" children (Greene, 2012). Greene's main message was on the surface an appealingly forgiving one: *children*, he repeated frequently, *do well if they can*. Beneath this mantra of faith in children's inherent desire to successfully comply with adult expectations, however, lies a corollary assumption. When children don't do well—when they interrupt the teacher or stare out the window during class or when they rage against pointless assignments or unfair punishments—it's not because they are choosing to disobey. It's because they have a deficit in their capacity for socially appropriate behavior. According to his "Bill of Rights for Behaviorally Challenging Kids,"

> Behaviorally challenging kids have the right:
> To have their behavioral challenges understood as a form of developmental delay in the domains of flexibility/adaptability, frustration tolerance, and problem-solving
> To have people—parents, teachers, mental health clinicians, doctors, coaches, everyone—understand that challenging behavior is no less a form of developmental delay than delays in reading, writing, and arithmetic, and is deserving of the same compassion and approach as are applied to these other cognitive delays. (Greene, n.d., para. 1–2)

In a popular YouTube video posted by Greene (2010), he compares the "earth-shattering philosophy" that "kids do well if they can" to the much more common assumption that "kids do well if they wanna." The text offered with the video reads:

> This is the most important theme of Dr. Greene's model: the belief that if kids could do well they would do well. In other words, if the kid had the skills to exhibit adaptive behavior, he wouldn't be exhibiting challenging behavior. That's because doing well is always preferable to not doing well.

Greene's approach emphasizes compassion and mutual respect. His Bill of Rights explicitly states his belief that blind obedience to authority is dangerous and that kids deserve to have their perspectives and concerns listened to and understood. Yet this formulation renders invisible the possibility of "behavioral challenge" as a form of deliberate, intentional, motivated, and meaningful resistance.

"Although neuroqueer subjects are often reduced to rigidity as a means of denying their rhetoricity," writes professor of English language and literature Melanie Yergeau (2018), "there is value in the clenched hand, in the anti-diplomatic gesture. As in, 'Fuck this. I'm autistic'" (p. 152). But as long as, to use Greene's (2010) formulation, "behavioral challenges [are] understood as a form of developmental delay in the domains of flexibility/adaptability, frustration tolerance, and problem-solving," then such challenging behavior can only be interpreted as a sign of individualized deficit in the capacity for responses that do not challenge (solving the problem, tolerating the frustration, adapting flex-ibly). The act of challenging a situation whose problems are beyond one's own capacity to solve is divested of meaning.

It's a Personal Decision That They Don't Think It's That Important

Kevin, a teenager diagnosed with Asperger's, was critical of such dis-cursive moves. I first met Kevin when he was 11. Curious and astute, he was at that time enthusiastic about his Asperger's diagnosis because he associated it with a community of so-called nerds that he'd found on the Internet. Over the years, however, he became more skeptical about the diagnosis. By the time of this interview, when he was 17, he had become quite wary of the way the Asperger's diagnosis was used to ascribe a lack of agency to those living under its description. He emphasized, instead, the importance of interpreting behavior as a deliberate choice. "This is how it is with a lot of things with Asperger's," he told me.

> When I was younger it was really hard for me to shower. Just because
>   it's such a monotonous thing to do. It still is, but I get it done anyway.
>   People think like: *oh, this person doesn't understand that it's important
>   to shower if you have Asperger's*. But no: it's a personal decision that
>   they don't think it's that important. They might fully understand how
>   it impacts them and be like, *well, if you're going to judge me based on
>   whether I'm showering, I don't want to be friends with you*. That's fair.
>   Same with any issue that a person with Asperger's might have. . . .
>   Like as an example—not me personally, I try not to curse in public,
>   but—someone could say: *People tell me not to curse in public but I
>   don't give a fuck, because if someone's gonna judge me for cursing then
>   I don't wanna be around them anyway*. And people will be like *oh,
>   that's because he has a social disability*—no it's fucking not! [Laugh-

ing] It's because they don't want to be around people who don't want
them cursing in public!

ELIZABETH: What if it becomes disabling?

KEVIN: Then you can address it psychologically, when it's a big issue
for someone. It's going to disable some people. Everyone's gonna
have some things they stand up for themselves on, even if it's bad for
them. But if it does get excessive, we can face it as a psychological endeavor. But not as Asperger's, just as *things*. Not just: *Oh, you're doing
this because you have "blank."*

Kevin, by this point in his life, had a long history of standing up for
himself on things that were bad for him. Intellectually gifted and desperate to go to college even when I met him as an 11-year-old (he treated
the University of Chicago business card I gave him with extraordinary
reverence), he had struggled his way through a series of school place-
ments and an unhappy period of homeschooling only to drop out of
community college after less than a year, deeply disappointed with the
quality of conversation he found there. He'd run away from home several times; he lived on the street for a while after the family he'd been
staying with cut off his Internet access. When I last saw him, he was
living with his mother, sporadically employed, dreaming of attending
a self-designed graduate program where he could research time travel
and change the world.

His mother, Laurie, a poet and activist with a vivid, intense demeanor,
struggled constantly with these same questions of how to explain her
son's troubles. How many of his travails came from having been a pre-
cocious kid understimulated by the material he was taught in school?
How much was a result of their explosive family dynamic—his absent
father, the screaming fights, her feeling of being constantly stretched to
the breaking point? How much was the Asperger's? How do you even
begin to pick these things apart?

LAURIE: Every once in a while, I see a flash, and I say OK, that's
definitely Asperger's, and you have to face it. But lots of times,
things he does that they call Aspergian and I wouldn't necessarily
call it Aspergian, and it could just be plain old stubbornness. . . .
For instance, with a teacher, if he'd say, *"Why do I have to do this,*

it's stupid"—what if it really is stupid? What if it really is five years
below his ability? Things like that.

People living with these new neurodevelopmental conditions, on the
border between self and disease, grapple constantly with what Brodwin
(2013) calls the "everyday ethics" of their interpersonal interactions. To
use the formulation from Allen's stepfather Fred, what is *the real*? And
what becomes of life experiences that are not accorded that ontological
status? Kevin and Laurie, and others in their boat, are "moral pioneers"
(Rapp, 2000), grappling with deeply significant philosophical questions in
the negotiations of their everyday lives. The discourse of individuals with
Asperger's syndrome as innocent machines, their decisions and behaviors
and communications as morally inert as a light switch, fails to capture the
social stakes of their interactions, the ways in which they are constantly
bound up in webs of needs and desires, both their own and others.

Both at Brookfield and outside of it, individuals with Asperger's syndrome are uniquely positioned to serve as the exemplars of a particular
brainhood: the brain as fixed, self-contained, and material, cordoned
off from the messiness of intersubjectivity and its moral valence. Their
behaviors can be interpreted as rigid, rule-bound, and mimetic, evoking the hardwired brain as a closed, fixed system. Repeatedly replicat-
ing their own behaviors and responses, they evoke certain ideals about
the scientific method and the contours of its products, as well as popular stereotypes about its practitioners. Exemplifying this model of the
psyche helps the students and their families to protect a small sanctuary
of consistent social space. It helps them acquire the tools they need to
develop their potential. And it provides an explanation that allows for
the creation of a little interpersonal distance, making conflictual moments more manageable. However, depicting the Asperger's students
as alienated from the social meaning that comes with moral accountability occludes their agency and conceals the stakes of their resistance.
And it makes no room for the complexities of their interpersonal entanglements, the many ways in which the stakes of their actions are co-
constructed between them and their interlocutors rather than inhering
entirely within their own innate characteristics.

The construction of what it means to have Asperger's syndrome
within the parameters of the Brookfield school system also constructs

what it means to be "psychiatric": as erratic, culpable, dangerous, and interpersonally engaged. It sequesters these messy fundamentals of human social life while casting them as less valued and less valuable. The resonance between the behaviors of people with each of these conditions—innocent but rigid and socially estranged in one case and unpredictable but adaptively, responsively human in the other—and the ontologies underlying the diagnostic systems within which each are classified—the hardwired and the malleable, the developmental brain and the psychiatric mind—give rise to a discourse in which these aspects of human experience are opposed, and seen as separable from one another. As we will see, these concepts have purchase well beyond Brookfield.

4

Hardwired

It's Not Neurochemical, It's Structural

I am sitting at a monthly meeting of the local chapter of the Asperger Support Network (ASPNET). ASPNET is a national organization that holds support group meetings in a number of major U.S. cities. Unlike many groups for people on the spectrum run by neurotypical facilitators, assumed to have expertise by way of their professional training, ASPNET meetings are planned and run entirely by and for adults who have been diagnosed, or who self-identify, as having Asperger's syndrome or a similar autism spectrum condition. Each meeting has some time for introductions and announcements, some time for attendees to problem-solve with the group about issues they may be facing, and then a discussion of a topic of general interest. The topic of today's discussion is medications, and the overall consensus is that they don't work very well.

"I don't want to take something to fix me. I'd rather work on things myself. This is who I am and I need to learn to live with myself the way I am," says Eduard, a young man in his mid-20s who is a regular attendee at these meetings. George, that week's meeting facilitator, speaks up to clarify. There are no medications that work directly to "fix" Asperger's, he notes, only medications for the depression and anxiety that arise from "all the depressing things about living with Asperger's! Because my understanding is, it's not neurochemical. It's structural, it has to do with brain structure."

On the face of it, George is just stating a known medical fact. Unlike many other mental conditions such as depression or schizophrenia, no medication has been found that can target the core symptoms of Asperger's syndrome or other autism spectrum disorders with which it is commonly grouped. But when George asserts that his condition is "structural" rather than "chemical," he is doing more than stating a fact about the treatments available for his condition. He is also invoking a complex and connotatively rich meaning system, an emerging cultural model that differentiates his condition—and himself—from other kinds of clinical conditions and those who struggle with them. It is a differentiation with powerful moral, practical, political, and aesthetic ramifications for George's identity.

In an influential investigation of sciences of the self and their impact on the identity of individuals, Nikolas Rose (2003, 2007) has chronicled the emergence of a "neurochemical self," profoundly influenced by the truth claims of the pharmaceutical industry:

> Individuals themselves and their authorities—general practitioners, nurses, teachers, parents—are beginning to recode variations in moods emotions, desires, and thoughts in terms of the functioning of their brain chemicals, and to act on themselves in light of this belief . . . and to see psychiatric drugs as a first line intervention, not merely for symptom relief but for ways of modulating and managing these neurochemical anomalies. (2007, p. 223)

Rose's analysis of contemporary biopower highlights the ways in which changes to the technologies through which we visualize, analyze, and act on the body—and, in particular, the brain that is understood to be its locus of self—connects to a broader set of sociopolitical imperatives. The availability of pharmaceuticals and the ways their effects are researched and marketed contribute to the expectation that "the active citizen must engage in a constant process of modulation, adjustment, and improvement in response to the changing requirements of the practices of his or her mode of everyday life" (Rose, 2003, p. 430). These assumptions are undergirded by a "neuromolecular" thought style: a reduction of larger organismic systems to small parts that can be studied separately from the wholes to which they belong (Abi-Rached & Rose, 2010) Neurochemical selves are characterized by ongoing liquid movement; by fluidity and flow, a constant change of shape around shifting parameters. As we saw in the previous chapter, such "psychiatric" personhoods are understood as malleable, responsive, and morally agentic in comparison to the fixed, innate, and faultless quality of developmental disability.

This mode of everyday life is well-captured by sociologist and political philosopher Zygmunt Bauman, who opens his 2000 book *Liquid Modernity* by quoting the *Encyclopedia Britannica*'s definition of *fluid*:

> This continuous and irrecoverable change of position of one part of the material relative to another part when under shear stress constitutes flow, a characteristic property of fluids. In contrast, the shearing forces within a solid, held in a twisted or flexed position, are maintained, the solid undergoes no flow and can spring back to its original shape. (p. 1)

This definition, he claims, "reads like a bid to deploy 'fluidity' as the leading metaphor for the present stage of the modern era" (p. 2), a stage characterized by "extraordinary mobility" and an absence of stable structures and bonds. Unlike the previous era of modernity, in which "the task confronting free individuals was to use their new freedom to find the appropriate niche and to settle there through conformity: by faithfully following the rules and modes of conduct identified as right and proper for the location," today "it is such patterns, codes and rules to which one could conform, which one could select as stable orientation points and by which one could subsequently let oneself be guided, that are nowadays in increasingly short supply" (p. 7).

At ASPNET, the fluidity of neurochemical selfhood and its association with mental, psychiatric, and/or emotional disorders were frequently evoked only to be rejected in favor of an alternative identification, what I call "neurostructural" selfhood. This counterdiscourse of the "neurostructural self" is oriented around the concept of developmental disability, its presumption of innateness and lifelong course, and its core domains of interest: learning, sensation/perception, attention, memory, information processing, self-regulation. In rejecting the demands for fluidity, flexibility and adaptation entailed in neurochemical selfhood, this counterdiscourse, of the solidity of the synaptic structure, functioned as a form of advocacy for the maintenance and recovery of local bonds. Here, I use the word *local* both in the sense of being rooted in physical space and in the sense of "local coherence" as a cognitive style: the emergence of meaningful phenomena out of consistent relationships between "stable orientation points" (to use Bauman's, 2000, phrase) within a system. As such, it functioned as a form of personal and political resistance; as advocacy for the consistent, permanent, and unchangeable; and as the articulation of a self that cannot be altered and still maintain its identity.

This chapter draws primarily on interviews and observations from the 4 months I spent observing and conducting interviews with participants at ASPNET meetings in and around Park City, a large metropolitan area a short distance away from Brookfield. After 8 months, I wrapped up my initial phase of fieldwork in Brookfield; I said my good-byes to the students and teachers at ASPEN and Valley View, to Sylvester and Annie, with promises to return for some follow-up fieldwork the following year. My soon-to-be-fiancé and I had moved to a little sublet in Park City so that I could do some participant-observation of the Asperger-specific programming at a medical school affiliated with one of the city's universities. I wanted to get a sense of the "medical model" of Asperger's syndrome in practice and figured that a medical center would be a good place to do that. Shortly before I arrived, however, the program that I had arranged to observe had gone through a reorganization of their staff and services, and the leadership no longer felt comfortable having an ethnographer present. There was some possibility I might be able to observe elsewhere in the clinic, but the arrangements were taking a bit of time. So I'd been cooling my heels in Park City for the time being and spending a lot of time with folks I met at various ASPNET support groups, where I'd gotten permission to observe and to recruit interviewees from both the executive director of the organization and the leaders of various local groups. In the process, I learned a great deal about the challenges faced by people with Asperger's and related conditions as they try to put together their adult lives.

Off the Cliff

The transition from adolescence into adulthood is a tricky time for many people on the autism spectrum. The expectation that they live independently, leaving home for college or for their own self-managed living space, removes many of the structures and supports that may have helped them during their childhood and adolescence. A study assessing social functioning in adolescents diagnosed with Asperger's syndrome, as compared to a group of adolescents diagnosed with conduct disorder, reported:

> Of the social impairments in AS [Asperger's syndrome] individuals, perhaps the most striking result is their profound lack of ability for independent living, given their intelligence and often good functioning in other areas. None of these normally intelligent young adults were considered by their parents capable of purchasing major items or engaging in leisure activities independently outside the home. Only a handful were able to travel at all independently, make any decisions about self-care, or even use the telephone. None had held down even a part-time job. (Green, Gilchrist, Burton, & Cox, 2000, p. 290)

Furthermore, the federal mandate to provide a "free and appropriate" education, which often includes services such as speech therapy, vocational training, and help with social and emotional learning as well as academics, ends after high school and a transition period. A 2015 National Autism Indicators Report from the AJ Drexel Autism Institute at Drexel University described the situation by coining the memorable phrase "the services cliff":

> Young adults with autism have a difficult time following high school for almost any outcome you choose—working, continuing school, living independently, socializing and participating in the community, and staying healthy and safe. To complicate matters, many of these youth begin their journey into adulthood by stepping off a services cliff. Access to needed supports and services drops off dramatically after high school—with too many having no help at all. (Roux, Shattuck, Rast, Rava, & Anderson, 2015; see also Roux et al., 2013)

A 2014 review of longitudinal follow-up studies on adults on the autism spectrum found that "adult outcomes in social integration and independence were reported to be mainly poor or very poor . . . with 50% or more of participants remaining fully or largely dependent on parents or carers and requiring significant support for education, living arrangements and employment" (Magiati, Tay, & Howlin, 2014). Those with higher IQ and stronger language ability tend to fare better. However, a 2012 review of outcome studies found that "as adults, many people with ASD, including those of normal IQ, are significantly disadvantaged regarding employment, social relationships, physical and mental health, and quality of life" (Howlin & Moss, 2012, p. 275; see also Howlin, 2000). In one study of 60 adults with autism, all of whom had been assessed with normal-range nonverbal IQ, most reported that they had never had a friend or any other close, reciprocal relationship, none were currently married, and most lived in situations where they had limited autonomy (Howlin, Moss, Savage, & Rutter, 2013; see also Gray et al., 2014, for similar findings).

I found it surprising—and perhaps you will as well—that the clever, articulate philosophers I met in Brookfield and then at these ASPNET meetings might have so much trouble. To an extent, the discrepancy is due to their being a different cohort: They had been diagnosed later than many of the participants in these studies and thus under widening guidelines, and many also had access to more services in their early developmental years, supporting better outcomes. But their situations were nonetheless often deeply precarious. Among the ASPNET attendees I got to know, their difficulties were often, for the most part, not large, grossly evident impairments but instead were with the micro: the fine, constant, tiny little choice points that constituted the texture of their daily lives and the challenge of negotiating these choices as autonomous, atomized agents.

"Asperger's is not a mental *disorder!* It's a *disability*—it's just that it's a disability you can't see," Doug, a 35-year-old ASPNET member, emphasized in our interview. I asked him about the difference between mental disorder and disability. "*Disorder* has such a negative connotation to it. Disability is a little bit more, like, someone has a learning disability—that person needs, just needs a little bit of help! So, people with Asperger's need a little bit of guidance with things that come easier to other people."

I asked him what kinds of things he needed guidance with. "Executive function issues that I have, just being able to pick *clothes* out, y'know—that look right, I have trouble with that, still. I know it sounds silly, but I still have that problem." There are a lot of considerations. "Is my shirt wrinkled? Is it too small, is it too large? Is it the wrong color for the occasion? Are the pants too short, or does it not go together? All that stuff!

All that stuff, you gotta worry about." Doug struggles with anything involving physical coordination; he couldn't tie his own shoes until he was a teenager, so he just wore shoes with Velcro for years. Sensory sensitivities make it hard for him to wear dress shirts with collars, even when his work demands it. He lives with his parents; before she left for a trip, his mother sat down with him, and they selected the clothes that he would wear to work while she was away.

The neuropsychological construct that Doug refers to earlier, *executive function*, refers to a set of abilities related to planning, decision making, judgment, and self-regulation, associated with various areas and connections within the prefrontal cortex of the brain. As a review in the journal *Current Directions in Psychological Science* puts it,

> various functions or abilities are thought to fall under the rubric of executive function. These include prioritizing and sequencing behavior, inhibiting familiar or stereotyped behaviors, creating and maintaining an idea of what task or information is most relevant for current purposes (often referred to as an attentional or mental set), providing resistance to information that is distracting or task irrelevant, switching between task goals, utilizing relevant information in support of decision making, categorizing or otherwise abstracting common elements across items, and handling novel information or situations. . . . it involves an *individual* guiding his or her behavior, especially in novel, unstructured, and nonroutine situations that require some degree of judgment. (Banich, 2009, p. 89, emphasis in the original)

Executive function is one of the areas frequently said to be compromised in autism spectrum conditions. Certainly, many people on the spectrum find it difficult to move fluidly through the range of consequential options one is confronted with on a daily basis in the course of living a life in which "novel, unstructured, and nonroutine situations" (Banich, 2009, p. 89) are the order of the day.

Doug is a tall fellow with a big, stretchy grin. He speaks with a pronounced lisp that accentuates the ways that he seems childlike, and distracts from the fact that he is also a wise and competent adult. He often gave both Eduard and me rides to the train from the ASPNET group, because neither of us had a car, and his playful warmth put me immediately at ease. But for a long time, he let people see very little of himself. "I was always very scared. Always very scared. And my way of dealing with it was to withdraw inside myself." He made it through school without any formal special education services by doing his best to fade into the background—a strategy that also left him with few social connections, mediocre grades, and a sense that he didn't really understand a lot of things. "Whatever I tried, I failed at it. I was very shy—very, very, very shy. It was like, it was very much like that I was present in the room, in class, or at school, but I really wasn't. So that part of my life was very—I was alone a lot, and it didn't go well, at all."

In college, he barely made it through, struggling in classes in which the expectation was that he would speak up for himself, ask questions, and self-advocate. "I was good with information type classes, things that you read from a textbook, study it, take a test. Information kind of classes, I did real well at. Classes that had to do with presentations, a lot of social interaction, I failed at." After college, he couldn't find a job—in 6 years, he only had one job, which he liked but lost after a year. He didn't have any friends—he had plenty of acquaintances, but the relationships never really transitioned into anything closer. "I think it was a lot of the social disabilities that I had. There's a lot of verbal, nonverbal, the cues, the behaviors—all the stuff like that was difficult for me." He never had a girlfriend, and as he watched family members get married, one by one, he asked himself again and again why it was so hard for him to do things that looked so easy for others. "My life was very, very, very down. I was very, very down. I felt like everything was *lousy*."

Around this time, Doug's parents met Eduard's sister-in-law at an event. They got to talking about Asperger's. *That sounds like Doug!* they thought. Doug went for an evaluation and was diagnosed with Asperger's. After the diagnosis, Doug started getting vocational services through an agency that works with people with disabilities and wound up getting hired, with the assistance of a job coach, at a small company where the founder has a family member on the autism spectrum. And he started going to groups at ASPNET.

The Asperger's diagnosis provided Doug with an explanatory narrative that helped him make sense of his life struggles. "I was relieved, and also concerned about what it meant," he told me. "Overall, I felt baggage was lifted off of me."

I asked him where that feeling of relief came from.

"A reason. A reason. A reason why I was the way I was." Knowing the reason has helped Doug figure out his next steps. "Now I at least know why everything's been hard. And I can take the steps, whatever steps I need to do to improve the things in my life that have caused so much despair." He chuckled, softening the bleakness of his words. "It made me feel that maybe there was light at the end of the tunnel. There was an explanation for all the stuff going on in my life."

Along with an explanation, and a sense of hope, ASPNET has given Doug a sense of purpose and a sense of community. "I think the diagnosis has allowed me to fulfill some of the things lacking in my life," he told me. "Being with others that have experienced similar things than I have made it a lot more comfortable. Being at these groups made me feel a lot more relaxed about it, not so confused anymore, and feel that while I'm learning about myself and trying to improve, I could help other people. There's tons of kids out there in their teens, that have [Asperger's], that have no support service whatsoever, don't know anything about ASPNET. If I can be just *this* much [help], then I'll feel very good that I did what ASPNET is trying to do."

I asked him what ASPNET is trying to do. "Building community, advocating for ourselves to get the things that we need, speaking for ourselves until we get what we need to handle living in this neurotypical world, which we find difficult to do." He told me the story of a teenager on the autism spectrum who had committed suicide. Would she have done so, he wondered, if she'd had access to a group like this? "We have to get chapters in as many places as possible. That's what I'm advocating. I'm not in the pity party anymore. I used to be: *Oh, woe is me.* I'm not, anymore." Instead, Doug has a shared cause. "Our cause is education, community—everything that ASPNET advocates. Everything that ASPNET advocates is what I advocate."

Everything That ASPNET Advocates

At ASPNET, people diagnosed with Asperger's syndrome and related autism spectrum conditions came together for the purposes of both mutual support and advocacy. Participants shared strategies for getting along in an often mis-fitting, ever-changing, and confusing world while also striving to develop a shared sense of their condition and its implications—a sense developed out of their own experiences and on their own terms rather than one handed to them by medical professionals.

A great deal of meaning-work took place in such spaces, spanning private experience and public representation. Members wrote books and blogs, and provided consultation to media outlets about the depiction of their contested condition. (At one meeting I attended, a very creative member even performed a one-woman courtroom drama she had written in which sensationalist media stereotypes about Asperger's syndrome—*"CYBER-CRIIIIIIIME!"*—were adjudicated and dismissed). Every once in a while, a screenwriter or movie star would show up at our grungy, linoleum-tiled meeting space seeking consultation on how to create realistic autistic characters. Participating in my research was, implicitly or explicitly, part of that process of advocacy around issues of representation.

Much like the Aspie communities of Brookfield, social life in ASPNET groups involved a lot of repetition, interpersonal uncertainty, and volatile emotion, and certain images, concepts, discursive systems, and fragments were introduced, echoed, charged with intense affect, and thus rapidly amplified. (If you like, if you'd like to get drunk while reading this book, you could drink every time somebody mentions Bill Gates's mother and her reproductive choices). They are therefore a rich source of what psychological anthropologist Claudia Strauss (2005) refers to as *social discourses*: explicit ideologies expressed through recognizable sets of ideas, jargon, and phraseology. The social discourses emphasized and elaborated at ASPNET helped participants organize their life histories, make sense of their present situations, and plan for their futures. They resonated consequentially within those enclosed meeting rooms—and outside of them as well.

Conceptualizations of Asperger's syndrome, the affected person, and the relationship between that were similar to those I heard at ASPNET also circulated through other spaces I observed that were similarly run by and for people on the autism spectrum for the purposes of community-building and self-advocacy. In particular, I also draw in this chapter on some interviews I conducted at an annual get-together run by and for people on the autism spectrum that I'll call Autspace. Unlike ASPNET, which was specifically geared toward people who understood themselves to have Asperger's syndrome, Autspace was explicitly defined as a place for *autistic* people, deliberately seeking to be inclusive toward the full range of people that the term autism can describe. There were therefore some significant differences between Autspace and ASPNET, in terms of both the people who attended and the nature of the discourses that were most prevalent there. However, a number of common themes also emerged in my observations and interviews in both spaces.

In both spots, Asperger's syndrome (and, often, autism as a whole) was often described as a difference in one's neurogenetic hardwiring. This metaphor was used to evoke an understanding of Asperger's much like we saw in Brookfield: as innate, fixed, and faultless, fundamentally differentiated from the socially and morally valenced mental health conditions that emerge out of tangled causal webs of interpersonal relationships. The metaphor of hardwiring also connoted a particular model of the self: as a fundamentally fixed and interconnected system from which no one part can be removed without radically transforming the nature of the whole, with Asperger's a determinative, pervasive, morally neutral, and often value-producing aspect of that system. As such, Asperger's was often explicitly defined against that which it is not: It is not a disease or illness, defined as entirely negative and separable from the affected person, and certainly not a mental illness, understood to be transient and arising from life experience. Instead, Asperger's is understood to be rooted in the physical givens of the body, the body is interpreted as a closed system that constitutes the self, and that self is experienced as vulnerable to annihilation if any of its fundamental elements are altered. This process of shared meaning-making provided narrative organization and a sense of community for often chaotic and isolated lives.

It's a Different Kind of Wiring

Katrin, a young woman I met through ASPNET, had been an awkward, introverted teenager. In eighth-grade study hall, she used to stare out the high classroom windows, calming herself by watching swaying treetops. Her classmates would stand behind her, encouraging her to jump to her death. Unsure of what to do to get them to stop, she would suffer in silence until she exploded with rage; then she got into trouble while her tormentors laughed from the sidelines. At the time, she believed that a separate part of herself, the part that was "Asperger Katrin," was to blame.

"When I was younger," she told me, "I really didn't understand Asperger's. I would always say there was Asperger's Katrin and Katrin Katrin. I felt like there was two parts of me, that there was some other person who was functional and who could live in the world and be normal. There was this other part of me that was keeping all that from happening. I really perceived them as, like, different spheres. The Asperger Katrin was like the evil twin, and the Katrin Katrin was the good twin."

Now a poised young woman in her mid-20s, Katrin has come to see herself in a more integrated way. "I don't see it like that anymore. There is no good and evil, and who I am is not evil." When I asked her to tell me how she would explain Asperger's today to someone who had never heard of it, she promptly replied: "I would say it's a neurobiologic difference in our minds. It's a different kind of wiring that makes it difficult for us to understand social cues and social interactions, and it also creates some sensory issues. I tend to react to loud noises and bright lights, some textures of food, clothing textures—things like that. But it's not a disease, and it's not an illness. It's a part of our personality and part of who we are."

Katrin has effectively summarized, here, the key points of the social discourse I am describing. The metaphor of "wiring," for Katrin, connotes her construal of Asperger's as a physiologically determined, morally neutral, inseparable and intrinsic aspect of how she perceives and processes the world and thus of who she is—both as an individual and as part of a "we." All these elements coexist within her conceptual schema of Asperger's, each entailing the others. But equally important, in her definition, is what Asperger's is *not*. I asked Katrin what she meant by "disease." What was she saying it *isn't*?

"Well, a lot of people, they think of autism and Asperger's, they think of disease. And when you have the word *disease*, you automatically have the word *cure*. There is no cure for Asperger's, and there is no cure for autism. You can't cure part of who a person is. You just can't. A disease is, by definition, something that makes you sick or incapacitated in some way. A disease is largely a negative word."

A disease, here, is something that can be removed from the affected person and something that is exclusively negative in its impact. Asperger's, on the other hand, is a difference that affects Katrin in a number of ways, some of which are good, some of which are bad, and many of which vary in their impact depending on the context. However, the way she talks about Asperger's tends to foreground its positive contributions, both to society, as a whole, and her own life, in particular. While she had been unable to keep a regular 9–5 job due to her difficulty navigating office environments, she had recently launched a career as a public speaker talking about her experiences on the autism spectrum and was in the process of writing a book on the subject. She was excited about the opportunities her condition had brought her. "For a long time when I thought of Asperger's, I could only think of how it negatively impacted my life 'cause that was the only effect I ever saw," she told me. "Now, all I see is how positively it impacts my life."

A Mac, Not a PC With a Virus

In addition to distinguishing autism and other neurodevelopmental disabilities from diseases, metaphors of wiring are also often used to differentiate these conditions, understood to be fixed, lifelong, and innate, from mental or psychological issues, understood to arise from life experience. At one ASPNET meeting, for example, the father of a young man diagnosed with Asperger's ventured a speculation that rather than there being a sharp line distinguishing those on the autism spectrum from "neurotypicals," perhaps we are all on the same "human spectrum." That week's facilitator, who was a charismatic and well-respected leader at ASPNET, firmly corrected him. "There really is a difference between people on the spectrum and those who aren't—it's in the brain, it's *wiring*." When the man retorted that perhaps all our neuroses are wired in too, the facilitator shook his head decisively. "Sometimes, people on the spectrum will develop problems that are psychological, as a result of what they've encountered. But the *difference* isn't."

The metaphor of computer operating systems is often used to highlight the contrast between conditions that are problematic intruders to a system and conditions that instead constitute the system itself. A 2015 post on Tumblr on "Mental Illness vs. Autism/Neurodiversity" by autistic blogger alice-royal begins by specifying that she is using the term *neurodiversity* to refer to "all personality disorders and developmental disabilities such as autism and ADHD" (para. 1). She then goes on to say:

> OK, so I've seen waaaaaaay too many posts lumping autistics in with mental illness groups and it's not cool because they are completely different.
>
> Mental illness is the equivalent of a PC with a virus. It is a working computer with its own personality that the virus has attacked and affected in its own unique way. My depression and anxiety are not a part of me and I do not like them and they change the way I think/feel/act from my 'normal'.
>
> Autism/other forms of neurodiversity are the equivalent of a Mac or Linux in a world of PCs. PCs think you're defective because you appear to be a PC with a virus but in reality you're a WHOLE OTHER OPERATING SYSTEM with all the strengths and weaknesses of any other, that just happens to be different from the majority of computers. But being a Mac is not a problem in the same way that being a PC with a virus can be a problem.
>
> Macs can get viruses—autistics can have mental illnesses, and people with mental illnesses can be autistic. But the two are not synonymous. We do not have the same terminology or community or anything. This doesn't mean that it's not okay to learn how to cope with mental illness or even be proud of it.
>
> Some people are treated for or recover from mental illness. You cannot change being autistic. You cannot treat being autistic. You cannot recover from autism.
>
> You cannot spend a lifetime trying to turn a Mac into a PC. You should learn how to protect and love both Macs and PCs.

The "operating system" metaphor emphasizes the ways in which "autism/other forms of neurodiversity" are pervasive, systemic, and neutral in their overall valence—not good or bad, just *different*. (I suspect the author may, as many do, have a preference between Macs and PCs, but it is not made explicit here). At the same time, they are also cast as productive and useful: Operating systems, after all, make computers usable for the many of us who don't know our way around a command line. A virus is far less valuable; a PC with a virus can, in fact, compromise the utility of other computers with which it comes in contact. In this respect, "forms of neurodiversity" are so different from mental illness that it is "not cool" to conflate the two.[1] Mental illnesses such as depression and anxiety are here depicted as unwelcome intruders that invade a system and compromise its function; autism, on the other hand, *is* the system itself. Consequently, *you cannot change it, treat it, or recover from it*; to do so is to attempt a fundamental alteration both impossible and unloving.

The metaphor of autism, and the group of similar conditions that it occupies, as the operating system of a computer defines the neurostructural self as a processing system, evoking the sort of neurocognitive domains associated with developmental disability and casting them as inherent and definitional elements of that self. Kent, a man I met at Autspace who was diagnosed with Asperger's syndrome at the same time his young son was, emphasized the extent to which such domains are "determinative of identity." He cautioned me in our interview against "medicalizing autism, and treating autistic people as broken nonautistic people, or nonautistic people with something wrong with them, like a broken leg or failing muscles or clogging lungs or whatever—any of these other medical diseases." Instead, he described "being an Aspie" as "probably as formative and informative of identity as being a man, being Jewish, having English as my mother tongue, being pretty close to the heterosexual end of the Kinsey Spectrum. Those are all attributes of me that determine who I am." When I asked him what it was about being an Aspie that made it more like being Jewish than like having a clogged lung, he replied: "Well, I think it affects the way that people think. I think it affects the way that people experience and express emotion. I think it affects the way memory works. I think it affects, even, the way we interact with our environment, through our senses. For that reason, I think it's much more determinative of identity than even various psychiatric conditions, maybe."

Kent's explanation for why "being an Aspie" is more like being heterosexual than it is like having a broken leg says a great deal about what he believes makes us the people we are. The kinds of functions that autism, as a neurodevelopmental disability, affects—expression, interaction, sensation, memory—connect the particularities of the person to the particularities of the world around them. These are understood to be "attributes of me that determine who I am" in a way that both psychiatric conditions and malfunctioning body parts are not.

The Box That Asperger's Comes In

Unlike conditions such as depression and anxiety, which hang together sensibly as folk categories, the cluster of characteristics that come together in neurodevelopmental conditions such as Asperger's are understood to be firmly grounded in the neurogenetic givens of physical human bodies, patterns that preexist our attempts to interpret and evaluate them. The correlation of traits that comprise the syndrome emerges out of objective realities of the body, not subjective judgments about what kinds of characteristics one might think would cluster together.

Talking to Marco, a man in his late 30s whom I met at an ASPNET meeting, I was struck by how much his identification with Asperger's, the reasons he found the syndrome compelling, were predicated on the ways in which the way the syndrome *contradicted* his intuitive sense of what characteristics are likely to coexist.

MARCO: It's tempting to describe Asperger's as a social deficiency and just leave it at that. But the lesson I learned last year when I started researching it, is that that's not all that you get with the box.

ELIZABETH: The box?

MARCO: The box that Asperger's comes in, it's not just social deficiency. You also get the sensory hypersensitivity, and all the other disconnected symptomology . . . in ways that you would never think are associated with each other.

ELIZABETH: What do you think causes all these things to correlate?

MARCO: Well it has to be a neurological level thing. It has to be something pertaining to the very basic functioning of the brain, how it's put together, that causes certain types of emotional level learning to happen in ways that do not in a neurotypical person.

Marco had read about Asperger's, but it had never occurred to him to investigate it further until he read an article that described it as involving not only social problems but also sensory hypersensitivities, which had troubled him since childhood. Only then did he feel he could talk with his family and partner about the possibility that he was on the autism spectrum—for the first time, the idea felt real, compelling. Incongruous characteristics are grouped through physiological, not subjective logics, and these logics have the ring of a robustly fixed and objective truth.

Because the set of characteristics associated with Asperger's are understood to correlate according to a fixed and interconnected physiological logic, this also implies that the valued and the disabling aspects of Asperger's travel as a set. When I asked Toby, a man in his 30s I met at Autspace, if he would, given the opportunity, go back in time and make it so that he had never had Asperger's, he responded:

> Realistically I'd have to give up all of the—like the way I make money now is that I can run analytical circles around everybody that I work with. And no matter how much they find me unpleasant or whatever, they always have to come back because they can't find anybody else to do what I can do, because it's just extremely narrow and in high demand. So realistically, I'd have to give up that, just the very specialized skills that I have and sort of the intelligence that was able to build those things, and that's a lot of who I am I guess.

The assumption Toby makes here, that giving up Asperger's would mean giving up not only his experience of social isolation but also his analytical thinking style, intelligence, and specialized skills (and thus "a lot of who [he is]"), is a common one. It depends on the presupposition that Asperger's is a linked series of traits in a consistent relation. We cannot selectively eliminate the troublesome parts of the condition and leave the elements we value. To acknowledge this is to prioritize the "realism" of objective physiology over wishful fantasy.

Just as autism is fundamentally interwoven into the person, per this view, it is also fundamentally woven into human history; autism has always been an important component of our genetic and neurological variation, which has provided humanity with many of our great and unconventional thinkers. Thus, one cannot eliminate autism from the human population without also eliminating the positive traits that go along with it by preemptively preventing the birth of idiosyncratic thinkers whose greatness is driven by such traits. This is a point frequently made by those concerned about efforts to develop a prenatal test for autism. Jake, a man in his mid-30s who led groups at ASPNET, said to me,

Well, what happens now, if they did find the cause for autism? The option is there that mothers would—let's say they: *Oh yeah, your son has this. Your son or daughter's gonna have this.* They may not want the baby. You know what I'm saying. We wouldn't have at least one president, you know, if it wasn't for Asperger's. We wouldn't have a lot of the great scientists. We wouldn't have a lot of people running the country. Some of the lucky ones who have the condition, and just happen to be—I'm thinking of Bill Gates, even though we don't know really in fact if he has it or not. But let's just take somebody like that. Let's say the mother had an abortion. You'd be depriving the world of Bill Gates possibly.

In evoking the possibility that extraordinary thinkers throughout history may have been extraordinary in multiple ways that would now fit under the rubric of Asperger's, this discourse emphasizes the multivalence of Asperger's: the capacity of the syndrome to describe not only vulnerabilities but also socially valued elements. At the same time, this emphasis on successful contributors—the great scientists, the "people running the country"—draws an implicit distinction between lives and attributes that are seen as productive and those that are not. Those who make use of such arguments against prenatal detection and prevention of their condition point out their own potential productivity and social value in order to make a convincing case for their right to survive and have a place on this earth—a right that often feels deeply threatened.

Eradicated From the Face of the Earth Forever

I first met Eduard at a bowling alley, where I was conducting participant-observation (by which I mean bowling, badly, in between conversations with my teammates) with a bowling league of adults on the autism spectrum that Jake had put together out of connections formed at a local ASPNET group. Supportive and kind, Eduard eventually became a good pal during my time in Park City. That first day, however, it took him quite a while to get up the nerve to speak with me. He first introduced himself to me by suggesting that I probably didn't want to talk to him. Once I pointed out that talking to people was exactly what I had come there to do, he started listing off other people in the group who I would probably rather be talking to instead. His expectation of rejection ran very deep.

When I told him about my project in a bit more detail, however, the conversation caught on. He started trying to explain how he felt when he heard people describe autism as something the world would be better off without. Within a few minutes, he was in tears. "Nobody wants to deal with people who have autism and Asperger's," he wept. "People say it's a horrible disease that needs to be eradicated off the face of the earth." In our interview several weeks later, he reiterated this idea:

> This is what gets me about Asperger's and autism these days, is that while there are other disabilities or diagnoses out there that people are good with living with, when it comes to Asperger's and autism, normal people feel that it is an absolute plague that must be eradicated from the face of the earth forever. And that really irritates me. . . . Look at all the celebrities going for Cure Autism Now.[2] They're trying to cure it because they want nothing to do with autism and what they fail to realize is we can't be cured, and maybe we don't want to be cured. We were born this way; please accept us for how different we are. But if you can't see that, clearly you don't want to know us. And you're just, you're just as bad as everybody else who judges us.

Eduard felt judged a lot. "When I meet people I'm always rejected," he told me. "Over time, it makes me extremely discouraged." He felt unwelcome at his workplace and worried that he was a burden on his family. Since his mid-teens, he had lived with his brother and sister-in-law, with whom he was in frequent conflict. "Even though they know I have Asperger's and my sister-in-law has helped me with the diagnosis and everything, I just don't feel like they can tolerate it. You know? I don't feel like my family could ever handle the fact that I was different from everyone." He hoped to live on his own someday—"I understand that people with Asperger's are going to have a hard time doing that, but I don't want to be one of those people who can't live independently"—but was also unsure about whether he would ever make enough money to afford rent (which was quite high in the area where he lived and worked) and wondered whether he could handle independent living. "If there's something I couldn't figure out, I can't just call someone for help. I don't know. If something breaks, I've gotta fix it, or if there's other issues that I'm not sure how to get out of—if I'm not ready for that, I'm not ready yet."

His deep and often thwarted desire to feel accepted informs his attitudes toward autism treatment. "I don't believe in treatment for autism and Asperger's," he told me, "because we are how we are—if the world can't live with it, it's too bad. So don't try to treat us, we are who we are, you've gotta live with it."

I asked him what he meant by "treatment"—what does he include under that term?

"I don't know. It could be anything. It could be pills, could be vaccines, I don't know. I just know that if people can't live with who we are, then the problem is not us, it's them." I asked him about speech therapy, psychotherapy. "I don't know because again, same thing, I don't think we should have to undergo any kind of treatment. They should recognize that that's how we're born and that's how we'll be. So I guess I'd say the same thing about that as I would about any physical form of treatment."

"What about social skills training, or, like, a social skills group?" I asked. At that point, things got more complicated.

"Well, OK. If I agree to any of this at all, I worry that it'll make me sound like a hypocrite, but I would like us to be able to get better social skills and be able to fit in with the outside world. But if that's a form of treatment, then I'm clearly a hypocrite and I'm sorry." Eduard did not want to be ideologically inconsistent. But at the same time, he yearned for help learning how to function better in his workplace, how to get along with other people better, and how to manage the unexpected challenges that might come with independent living. Interventions on his physical body, on the other hand, posed a different kind of threat. "Physical treatment is obviously a blatant attempt to either try to rid the world of autism spectrum disorders or try to rid the world of people with it. Either way, they're like: *Well, we can't live with this, you've gotta do something about this guy, we can't live with them.*" Intervention on the physical body, especially intervention that sought to take something away from the system that made Eduard who he is, threatened him with annihilating rejection. Removing such a constitutive piece from the system obliterates the whole.

An Organ That Never Stands Still

The discourse of tension between neurochemical and neurostructural understandings of the self, predicated on commonly held and institutionally entrenched assumptions about the relationship between mental health problems and developmental disability, is pervasive and powerful. However, it is increasingly destabilized by new models of the brain-in-the-world. Recently, a number of scholars have claimed that the dominant mode of neuro-selfhood is no longer neurochemistry but *neural plasticity*, characterized by a greater openness to the environment and potential for deeper change. Neurochemical modulation, for all its fluidity, is always constrained by the structure of the synapses through which these chemicals flow—just as the neurochemical discourse of the psychiatric exists, as I have shown, always in tension with the neurostructural discourse of developmental disability. Plasticity, on the other hand, encompasses both; it is the language of the *neurodevelopmental*, the innate and robust brain in interaction with the world over time. The kind of change which neural plasticity evokes, the arenas that it opens to intervention, are far more fundamental and expansive.

In his 2016 ethnography *Plastic Reason: An Anthropology of Brain Science in Embryogenetic Terms*, anthropologist and historian of science Tobias Rees describes the shift as follows:

> What was at stake was a shift from a conceptualization of the brain— the human—as a neurochemical machine largely determined in its basic design, fixed in its being, toward a conceptualization of the brain—the human—as a ceaselessly emerging cellular organ, an organ that never stands still, that is defined by an irreducible openness. At stake was a shift from neurochemistry to plasticity. (p. 8)

Plastic Reason tells the story of Alain Prochiantz, a maverick researcher who became first a pariah, then a paradigm-setter, for his insistence that "in truth, the brain is undergoing a constant renewal. There is nothing that is stable" (p. 195). The shift is mightily resisted by old-school scientists, stewing in their sea of wires, for whom it is a loss of a whole way of life, the sacrifice of a neurological ethic characterized by a logic of the self as "fixed and immutable."

Rees (2016) finds this state of transition to be thrilling, liberating, an invitation to a social scientific exploration of "an in-between, irreducibly open state" (p. 236). On the other hand, in her 2010 piece "The Plastic Brain: Neoliberalism and the Neuronal Self," sociologist Victoria Pitts-Taylor suggests "caution in celebrating plasticity as inherently liberating" (p. 639). In an analysis of popular science writing on the subject of brain plasticity, she warns that "the development of plasticity discourse is highly compatible with the neoliberal pressures of self-care, personal responsibility, and constant flexibility" within a "competitive field in which one's willingness to let go of sameness, to constantly adapt, and to embrace a lifelong regimen of work on the self (and on one's children) are the keys to individual success" (pp. 640, 644). She argues for ethnographic investigation of the uptake of these discourses, pointing out that "we cannot assume that the neoliberal construction of subjects in neuroscience, medicine, and the public sphere is wholly successful; whether or not people actually relate to their brains in the ways they are encouraged to relate to them is a matter needing ethnographic attention" (p. 640). Looking ethnographically at the specific nuances and patterns of uptake and interpretation of neuro-discourse is especially important given that these discourses often organize people into groups according to sets of propensities that are relevant to their interpretation of such discourse. The diagnosis of autism, for example, tends to aggregate those for whom a lifetime of open-endedness, change, and transition is a pretty unpleasant prospect.

Neuro-philosopher Catherine Malabou (2008) has argued that the affinity between discourses of neurological self-fashioning and imperatives of global capitalism is better referred to as flexibility than plasticity. Flexibility is docile; plasticity, on the other hand, can give shape as well as receive it; it has the capacity to explode form as well as to hold it. The brain's capacity for plasticity, she argues, is potentially revolutionary; many of the existing discourses around plasticity, on the other hand, merely work to naturalize models of capitalist society. "*What should we do so that the consciousness of the brain does not purely and simply coincide with the spirit of capitalism?*" she asks in *What Should We Do With Our Brains?* (p. 12, emphasis in the original). "When does openness to the future simply become pliability and compliance—and how can one resist such an appropriation?" Nima Bassiri (2016, para. 13) similarly asks at the end of his review of *Plastic Reason*.

The concept of plasticity carries complex, multiplicitous sets of entailments and potentialities. What form they take, what kinds of forms they offer, what they solidify into, what they hold together, and what they explode all transpire within particular settings where they are taken up in practice. On one hand, the kinds of neuroscientific endeavors associated with plasticity offer a potential corrective to the oft-observed perils of neuro-reductionism, in that they invite serious consideration of environmental influence, often implying that the brain is itself designed to expect and deal with certain types of social and interpersonal engagement. They offer a developmental framework, in which the brain grows dramatically throughout life in interaction with environmental stimuli. They invite us to a consideration of the brain-in-the-world, in which our existence does not end at the edge of our skull or our skin but could perhaps be extended to the entire body and out to our material and social ecologies (Pitts-Taylor, 2016).

And, yet, this expansion of our openness, our presumed vulnerability and ability to benefit and suffer from the stimulation and stress that comes our way, is being investigated in a context that has historically been very thoroughly focused on the pathologies of individual bodies. The expansion of neuroscience into broader social, interpersonal, environmental terrain is often followed by the constriction of that new territory back into familiar forms, accessible through existing technologies and compatible with existing funding mechanisms (e.g., see Rose & Abi-Rached's, 2013, account of the history of social neuroscience). What are the consequences of this pattern of expansion and constriction over time? Without pushing the metaphor too far, it seems relevant to consider the fact that the most enduring legacy of plastic may not be its capacity to take form or to give form, but its propensity to survive subdivision into tiny little pieces, its capacity to become *microplastic*—and so to flow, through waterways, up food chains, and into the bodies of living creatures. Plasticity discourse, too, takes place within systems that subdivide us.

Bauman (2000), throughout *Liquid Modernity*, frets about the possibilities for collective resistance within a society taught to reinterpret social troubles as idiosyncratic, private concerns:

> Given the nature of today's tasks, the main obstacles which urgently need
> to be examined relate to the rising difficulties in translating private prob-

lems into public issues, in congealing and condensing endemically private troubles into public interests that are larger than the sum of their individual ingredients, in recollectivizing the privatized utopias of "life-politics" so that they can acquire once more the shape of the visions of the "good society" and "just society." (pp. 51–52)

A personal, metaphorical, aesthetic rehabilitation of wires, that is deeply lived, shared, and strategically amplified, is one way to resist. At ASPNET, the confession, display, and discussion of private worries are rooted in a discourse of bodily similarity that assumes the presence of both deep commonality and significant difference. Through this linking of individual particularities of embodiment with social and interpersonal collectivity, new relationships transform states of atomized isolation.

"That's how I made a friend!" Doug told me. "Before Eduard—I had *nobody*. I had *nobody*." Eduard has become Doug's first true friend, and he cherishes their relationship. The fact that they are both on the spectrum made it easier to connect, although it is not something they talk about much, and Doug can see that it affects them in different ways. "The fact that we both have Asperger's syndrome made it easier. You know, we're different. He likes video games, I don't like video games that much. So it's different, but I think the A. S. [Asperger's syndrome] filled a void, I guess. But that's my first friend! And before that: disaster. Everything, disaster."

Doug's connection with Eduard has expanded his world. Before he became friends with Eduard, he barely knew how to drive: All his driving experiences had involved his father yelling at him from the passenger's seat, making Doug so petrified he could barely see where he was going. Now, he told me, "I did it! I started to go out by myself. I found ways to do it without going on highways. And I take the same route to his house all the time, and I keep doing that all the time. So repetition has been very good to me. If I do something over and over and over again, I'm more comfortable with it." New connections are formed and maintained through the opportunity and motivation to repeat the same old routes.

"Even NT's [neurotypicals] have problems with change, and the problem's more acute as far as handling changes – more acute with people on the spectrum," Jake told me in our second interview. He was working hard to learn how to adapt to change. The workplace where he had held the same entry level job for the past 14 years was going through a reorganization, and he found the experience very stressful. "It's the on-the-spot changes that's most troubling with me. I can't speak for anybody else, but for me, it's all the surprise." He credited his ability to cope to his knowledge about Asperger's. "I'm not saying that life is great, but I'm doing better because I know how to manage it. I know what it is. I know how to manage it, and that's the important thing. I'm learning to smile. People like me a lot more. I'm talking to people, making small talk." But these changes are only surface-deep. "I can't go change my genes. I can change these jeans" he joked, gesturing at his pants, "but I can't change my genetic makeup. There's not much I can do with it."

"That's how it is," I replied.

"That's how it is," he agreed. "We're here. Deal with us. Deal with us."

The politics of the neurostructural self use the materiality of the biological brain and the inherence of the genetic blueprint as an argument for acceptance, and against the expectation of infinite flexibility and adaptation to change associated with neurochemical selfhood. In the process, this approach opens new possibilities for a form of resistance that is simultaneously individualized and collective, reinforcing consistent local connections against the constant pressure toward their dissolution. At the same time, it takes up a notion of the body as a closed system risking annihilation by external impingement and risks separating value-producing qualities from aspects of developmental difference that are not so generally seen to be productive. In these ways, its vision of the self as a closed neurogenetic circuit is circumscribed by the clinical science on which it is founded—a project driven by the very agendas of separation and elimination that the proponents of this discourse seek to resist.

5

The Pathogen and the Package

A World in Which Suffering Because of Autism No Longer Exists

I am sitting in an auditorium at the 8th International Meeting of the International Society for Autism Research—IMFAR, for short.[1] It is one of the largest of the annual autism conferences, dedicated entirely to scientific research. Each day of the conference opens with a keynote address, which is itself opened by introductory remarks from one of the foundations funding the conference. Today is the opening day of the conference, and these introductory remarks are provided by Geraldine Dawson, chief scientific officer of Autism Speaks.

In her 20-minute talk, Dawson lays out the strategic planning process and resultant strategic plan for Autism Speaks: making comprehensive medical evaluation and medical comorbidities a part of standard diagnostic workups for autism, looking at gene/environment interactions, translating genetic and biological findings into clinically useful tools for risk assessment and drug discovery, developing treatments of immediate benefit, effective dissemination and funding of empirically validated treatments, the creation and maintenance of biorepositories and bioinformatics, and being "innovative and nimble" in the rapid funding of high-risk, high-impact projects. The message is clear: As much as possible, let us focus our gaze on the molecular body, where truth can most efficiently be found and interventions most effectively targeted.

Autism Speaks was founded in 2005 by Bob and Suzanne Wright, grandparents of a child with autism, out of the merger of three smaller organizations, the most well known of which was Cure Autism Now. Over the next decade, the organization became a major player and influential force in the funding of autism research, with the mission of "funding global biomedical research into the causes, prevention, treatments and a possible cure for autism" (Diament, 2016, par. 6). It also became the subject of significant critique: for allocating so many resources toward prevention and cure at the expense of supporting autistic individuals and their families in a better quality of life, failing to include autistic people in positions of power within the organization, and consistently using rhetoric that cast autism as antithetical to a full and good life (Broderick & Ne'eman, 2008; Schultz, 2017; Stevenson, Harp, & Gernsbacher, 2011).

In her opening remarks, Dawson is clearly being careful to avoid re-inforcing this perception. "Persons with autism spectrum disorders are at the heart of everything we do," she tells the audience. "They are our True North, to which we point our compass." She reviews the Mission and Vision of the organization: their vision is "a world in which suffering because of autism no longer exists." I am struck by the wording, its deliberate delicacy: It is the *suffering because of autism*, not the people with autism or even the autism itself, that would no longer exist in the world this organization seeks to bring into being.

But there is a curious tension between the practices of the organization and its mission: "suffering because of autism" takes place outside of the cells and molecules where she recommends we look to find it and fix it. Suffering because of autism happens when a mother cannot connect and share an emotional experience with her child; it happens when that child cannot tell their mother what they want and need and when they resort to doing things that make them hurt more—head-banging, biting. It happens when they stand outside a circle of their peers, wishing to join in but unable to do so; it happens when they grow up and cannot get a job and then cannot pay for a place to live. We suffer because of autism because we are beings that suffer, not just a collection of molecules and genetic patterns, and that suffering happens because of problems between people, not only because of things that happen within a body. But the mission here is to find "suffering because of autism" in the molecular, biological body. The process requires a great deal of interpretive, imaginative, and analogical work.

Divided Medicalization

In *The Body Multiple: Ontology in Medical Practice*, ethnographer and philosopher Anne-Marie Mol (2002) depicts how medical settings simultaneously construct multiple versions of diseases sharing the same name; these multiplicitous entities are then made to cohere through a variety of institutional practices. Mol herself refrains from commenting on the consequences, beneficial or harmful, of these processes, calling for further ethnographic work that addresses that question in particular. Autism is a particularly generative site to answer this call. As medical anthropologist Sharon Kaufman (2010) has observed, autism is a particularly "mutable object of knowledge, a protean disease category" (p. 8) that is fluid in its form, boundaries, and contents and that reflects the uncertainties of multiple areas of life and knowledge production (see also Verhoeff, 2012). Autism itself has no physical presence outside of patterns of phenomena through which it can be creatively "traced" (Fitzgerald, 2017). There are no biomarkers consistently linked to autism—no lab test that can detect it, no imaging technique that can visualize its contours. It shows up in sociality, in behavior, in language. Locating autism in the physical body is thus always a process of representation and inference. We can locate genes in the body that are linked to some manifestations of autism for some people; we can observe consistent patterns of behavior and assume that they arise out of some underlying process in the body that we have yet to detect. When we conceptualize autism as a phenomenon arising within the body, our understanding of autism is always profoundly shaped by the metaphors through which we imagine its potential embodiment.

The category of autism has been expanding through a time of transition within psychiatric science, during which an older and newer paradigm have both been active, intersecting and overlapping with each other in complex ways, producing two different, and overlapping, models of autism. In many contexts, autism is depicted like a *pathogen*: a hostile invader of a closed system, exclusively negative in its impact, that compromises its health and integrity—something to be defended against, kept out, gotten rid of. However, shifts toward grounding psychiatric diagnosis in data from neuroscience and genetics are producing a different kind of autism: autism as a *package* of interlinked traits, through which the affected person interfaces with the world around them and which therefore may be valued or devalued depending on the context within which they manifest. The next two chapters of this book examine how these two models coexist and, in particular, what happens when the package comes to be represented and dealt with as a pathogen.

I refer to this process as "divided medicalization." Divided medicalization is a process of expansion and constriction that occurs when a condition is delineated under one knowledge production system expansively, containing a wide range of attributes and meanings (in this case, as a neurogenetic package) and through another in a more constricted way, containing only a subset or a transformation of those meanings (in this case, as a pathogen). When these two systems cooperate, aspects of lived experience are evoked and then occluded, expelled, collapsed, or deformed. People living under those descriptions thus live under a contradictory and ambivalent system of meanings.

A Perfect Description of Me

"Getting diagnosed was probably the best thing that happened to me." Lana is a willowy blonde in her mid-20s, with an unsettlingly direct, unwavering gaze. She is arrayed in a riot of bright colors, from the wildly assorted hues of her clothes to the neon-green headphones she uses to block out excess noise to the bright blue rubber ball she clenches and unclenches in one hand while talking to me. The sensory input from all these sources helps her to keep her nervous system in balance. "It just opened me up to this whole other community of people, and it helped me know myself so much better through learning about autism and meeting other autistic people. And I have a lot more self-confidence now, too, because I understand how I am."

I am sitting with Lana at Autspace. She is being very generous in spending some of this time with me because it's one of the few chances she has to meet up in-person with the community of autistic activists that she spends the rest of the year communicating with online. When she's done talking to me, she's going to go meet them at the pool.

Lana tells me that she likes being autistic, though she knows that not everyone does. And then she is careful to qualify:

> Sometimes when I say something like that, or when other people say something like that, some people will misconstrue that as saying: *oh, well, being autistic's all fun and games. And it's all a happy party, and I have no challenges, and I need no help.* And they think that we're whining if we ask for accommodations. *Well, you like your autism so you don't need an*

accommodation. No, that's not true. My autism is a part of me whether it's good, bad, or indifferent and it's all three at different times and different ways. There's a lot of elements of autism that I'm thankful for, that I think really help me, and then there's other parts of it that aren't positive or negative, but they're just part of my personality. They're what make me, me. And then there's a lot of stuff that is extremely challenging and disabling. And maybe I'd be happier without certain elements, but I know that it's a whole package.

Lana spent much of her adolescence seeing therapists and other mental health professionals, but the diagnoses they used to explain her distress—depression, obsessive-compulsive disorder, Tourette's syndrome—only addressed small, problematic pieces of her experience. None of them explained the things that mattered to her about herself: her obsession with her art, her inability to remember faces, her difficulty making friends and connecting with romantic partners, or the intensity with which she perceived the world—colors alluringly bright, tastes so strong and textures so harsh that she can eat only a limited range of foods without gagging. None of them covered "the whole package." None of them explained why she was the way she was. One day, however, while searching the Internet, she started reading about Asperger's syndrome—and she felt a shock of recognition.

"I was like, 'Oh, my God. This is a perfect description of me.' And I read a lot on the Internet and then I told my parents and gave them some stuff to read and they were like, 'Wow, this really is you. How come nobody we took you to ever saw this?' I think we were all kinda mad." Lana successfully sought out a formal diagnosis from a neuropsychologist who specialized in autism spectrum disorders:

I wanted to learn more about myself. I'd never had a neuropsych evaluation done. Never had any sort of testing or anything like that done. You know, I'd been to lots of therapists and psychiatrists, but nobody ever gave me a piece of paper that had any formal diagnosis on it. Nobody did like a full, like, "These are your cognitive strengths and these are your attention things." [I said]: "Just test me for everything across the board. I want to know myself better." [The neuropsychologist] wrote a big 15-page paper, did all of the studies and took a family history and all that, and it was painfully obvious to her that I was on the spectrum . . . she couldn't believe that none of [the prior therapists] saw it.

Lana got to know herself better through an increasingly common experience for youth who are perceived, or who perceive themselves, to fall outside of the norm: neuropsychological testing that assesses core perceptual, interpretive, attention, and self-regulatory processes along spectrums that range from extreme weakness to extreme strength. Note the inclusiveness of this evaluation, as Lana appreciatively describes it: Rather than focusing on a select group of symptoms, as her prior therapists had done, Lana's neuropsychological diagnostician did a "full" assessment that tested for "everything across the board"—cognitive strengths as well as weaknesses, "attention things" (not just attention problems). Through this new knowledge, these standardized measurements of cognition and attention that claim to comprehensively map the mechanisms determining Lana's experience of the world around her, Lana came to know herself. And the self she came to know was autistic.

Through this experience of identification, Lana became politically active in a way she had never been before. "I've never really been, like, an activist or a political person. I didn't even vote for the first time until this past year, because I could never make up my mind about anything" Lana told me. "And for the first time, I was enraged that people were being treated badly, and that people needed *this*, and they needed *this*, and that wasn't happening because of *this*. We're spending, I started learning, millions of dollars looking at genes and causation, but there's people here now that need help now, and less than 1% of all autism funding is going to actually helping people. It's all going to potentially maybe helping future people, but also potentially eliminating them, and also perhaps harming them. We don't know yet." Now, she works alongside other autistic people to advocate for private, state, and federal funding to be diverted away from biomedical research into preventing or curing autism, away from trying to pinpoint genetic risk factors for autism that might lead to prenatal testing and preventative abortion and instead toward helping autistic people have a better quality of life. "I think that autistic adults, and even children, are the people to ask about what's best for autistic people, because we know what it's like. And things are being decided without asking us."

Lana gets a lot of criticism, from others in the extremely broad and diverse community of people dealing with autism spectrum disorders, for her claim to know what is best for autistic people based on her own experience. For the parents of a severely disabled autistic adult who cannot speak, dress themselves, or go to the toilet unassisted, it is often hard to make sense of this articulate, college-educated young woman, and others like her, arguing passionately against a cure for autism, marshaling rhetoric about eugenics and the need for genetic diversity. *You're not autistic*, she's been told, even though she has an in-depth diagnostic evaluation that says she is. But Lana has learned that the commonalities between her and other autistic people run deeper than the tremendous differences that are visible on the surface.

"There are things I can relate to about just about any autistic person that I meet or who I hear about," she told me. "Even an autistic child that is, like, 3 years old and maybe doesn't talk at all, I could relate to him, even though I wasn't him when I was that age. Because our *brains* are more similar to each other than they are to other people, I think, even within the broad diversity of the spectrum. OK, some of us talk and some of us don't. Some of us work and some of us don't. Some of us make friends and some of us don't—but those are almost superficial differences. They seem so important, but they're not."

It's a remarkable statement: that similarities between brains are a deeper and more important indicator of common ground than whether one can talk (let alone what one says), whether one can hold a job (let alone what one does for a living), whether one makes friends (let alone who those friends are). In making this statement, Lana is drawing on a lived sense of experiential kinship with others whose cognitive processing style, sensorium, and overall approach to the world feels similar to hers—the kind of "mediated kinship" observed by Rapp and Ginsburg (2001). But she is also drawing on a form of more experience-distant scientific expertise that places objective physiological similarity ahead of socially co-negotiated and subjective interpretations of lived experience when determining what the word *autism* means.

In 2013, the fifth edition of the *Diagnostic and Statistical Manual of Mental Disorders* (*DSM-5*; American Psychiatric Association, 2013) radically changed the diagnostic nomenclature for autism, combining all the separate categories of "pervasive developmental disorder" (including Asperger's syndrome) into a single diagnostic term: "autism spectrum disorder." This change had been in the works since the beginning of the 21st century, part of a broader move away from categorical, symptom-based diagnoses and toward a reconceptualization of disorders as continuous spectrums dictated by neurobiology. A 2011 article in the *American Journal of Psychiatry* written by the chair and vice-chair of the DSM-V Task Force explained that "the proposal for a single 'autism spectrum disorder' category that would include the current DSM-IV diagnoses of autistic disorder (autism), Asperger's disorder, childhood disintegrative disorder, and pervasive developmental disorder not otherwise specified was born from data suggesting that these disorders share a pathophysiological substrate" (Kupfer & Regier, 2011, p. 2). This foregrounding of pathophysiological similarity reflects the increasing primacy of physiological etiology within a diagnostic classification system that is shifting away from exclusive categories and toward broad and inclusive continua, informing Lana's emphasis on commonalities between herself and other autistic people. As she says, although their lives may be very different, their *brains* are similar. The sweeping nature of these claims to kinship is supported by the development of a classification system that is based more on neurological and genetic physiology than subjective or social manifestations.

Lana's identity is thus intricately intertwined with cognitive, medical, and psychiatric science. She is an artist; she is an activist; she is the one who is always dressed in rainbow colors; but underlying and explaining all these attributes is the neurological makeup that makes her who she is. It is a system that can only be fully known through the interventions of clinical expertise. But Lana's relationship to science is as contentious as it is intimate, troubled by a conflict that lies at the core of such diagnostic identities. Clinical neuroscience, with all its explanatory power, gave Lana her sense of autistic personhood. Now, as she watches millions of dollars pour into researching prevention and cure while autistic children die in restraints in overcrowded classrooms and adults wait on endless lists for supported housing, Lana fears that the same process of knowledge production that illuminated her way of being is simultaneously working to destroy it.

Lana and her fellow young adults in the nascent autistic self-advocacy movement have come of age during a time of paradigm shift in psychiatric diagnosis. Conditions such as depression or obsessive-compulsive disorder were, for many years, conceptualized as discrete disease entities, sets of problems that seemed to hang together into coherent syndromes that could be envisioned as separate from the particular lives and bodies within which they manifested. Such a framework organized and motivated responses geared toward the elimination of these conditions, restoring the person to his or her original healthy self. However, Lana's sense of self has developed in the context of a newer and increasingly prevalent approach to psychiatric evaluation and diagnosis, what I refer to as the *neurodevelopmental turn*. In schools, as we have seen, the special education system teaches students to identify with their own thoroughly assessed capacities for learning, attention, emotion regulation, and social cognition, expanding the category of "neurodevelopmental disability" to a wider and wider range of developmental trajectories whose origins are understood to be innate. Meanwhile, within psychiatry, the most powerful figures in the field have spent the past two decades advocating for an overhaul of psychiatric diagnosis along the same lines.

The Neurodevelopmental Turn

In 2011, the website of the National Institute of Mental Health (NIMH, 2011) announced that "mental disorders are increasingly viewed as neurodevelopmental disorders in one way or another" (para. 13). This is to say, mental disorders are increasingly understood to originate within the brain, as propensities present in our genetic makeup, latent potentialities there from the very beginning of life. They manifest over time in abnormalities in universal brain functions, such as learning, attention, memory, and self-regulation, through which we know and engage with our world. Their contours are determined not by commonsense consensus about what kinds of experiences comprise a disorder but by patterns of correlated findings across levels of analysis: among cellular, neurological, genetic, and behavioral data, which may or may not correspond to our current categories of experienced impairment. These are generated out of scientific initiatives that seek to map complete and comprehensive systems thought to make us who we are: the circuit diagram of the human brain, the blueprint of the human genome. Developmental disorders, once marginalized within psychiatry, are at the center of this shift, and autism, as it morphs from a symptom to a spectrum, is its flagship condition.

This new approach to diagnosis is producing a different sort of diagnostic construct from the disease entities produced under the previous system. They are less like pathogens and more like—as Lana says—"a whole package." Rather than producing conditions that are exclusively negative, these new diagnostic constructs are *multivalent*: They contain elements that are wanted, elements that are unwanted, and elements that are neither, or both, depending on the context. Rather than producing conditions that are separable from and even antithetical to the personality of the person affected, they are producing conditions that are *identitarian*: They feel like a constitutive element of who we are as people in the world. Rather than producing conditions that breach the boundaries of bodies to then dwell within them or travel between them, they are producing conditions that are *worlded*: They exist in a complex and co-constitutive relationship with the world beyond the person, connected through experiences and practices that are irreducibly social, sensory, and aesthetic.

However, the new expansive quality of the diagnostic entities produced through this approach to diagnosis—their way of encompassing both the beautiful and the bothersome of human experience, their reach beyond the borders of the body into our perceptions and pleasures and social relationships—becomes constrained within clinical settings dedicated to identifying, containing, and eliminating problems-as-pathogens through closely managing the boundaries of both bodies and social spaces. While developmental disorders have long been considered fixed and incurable, in many cases motivating responses of accommodation, appreciation, and support, the research agendas driving the neurodevelopmental turn are motivated by the possibility of a very different response: presymptomatic identification and correction of developmental trajectories considered to be pathological. If we can learn to detect disorder in the body before it manifests as subjective, experiential distress, the theory goes, we can more effectively intervene to *prevent* those problems from developing.

In a moment when the nature and contours of diagnostic entities are in dramatic flux, however, this agenda raises an unresolved question: Presymptomatic detection and prevention of *what*? Clinical discourses of detection and prevention continue to treat autism as if it were an entirely negative phenomenon that could easily be separated from the affected person; meanwhile, the science undergirding these intentions, increasingly privileging objective observations of correlation rather than subjective consensus about impairment, is producing an autism that is lived in a way far more complex. In a time of increasing enthusiasm for universal autism screening (e.g., Mandell & Mandy, 2015) and for the identification of biomarkers that are thought to allow such screenings to proceed with greater efficiency and accuracy (e.g., Yusuf & Elsabbagh, 2015), what might appear to be a philosophical question has significant practical import.

I Crumpled Up Autism and Put It in the Garbage

Autism has a long history of being metaphorically depicted as a hostile intruder. As Emily Martin (1994) has vividly illustrated, the image of the body as a walled fortress under siege by foreign entities, malevolent invaders that would destroy it if they were allowed to be victorious, has long been a powerful organizing metaphor within American medical practice. Such militaristic rhetoric, as critical disability theorist Anne McGuire (2016) vividly illustrated in her book *War on Autism: On the Cultural Logic of Normative Violence*, is especially prevalent in the case of autism (see also Broderick, 2010; Broderick & Ne'eman, 2008). Autism is also frequently depicted through metaphors of confinement—fortresses or cocoons from which a child struggles to emerge—or through theories about contamination or penetration by foreign elements, such as poisons or toxins. Such metaphors organize stories about autism as fundamentally antithetical to the affected person.

During my fieldwork, I spent some time attending conferences of organizations within what is sometimes referred to as the "biomedical" or "biomed" movement in autism—those who seek to define and treat autism as a medical illness amenable to the kind of medical treatment that detects and remedies other bodily problems. Groups such as Generation Rescue, Talk About Curing Autism, AutismOne, and the Autism Research Institute (formerly Defeat Autism Now!) bring together parents, practitioners, and researchers who believe that autism is not a neurogenetic, innate, and lifelong disability but a "whole-body disorder" implicating the gut, immune system, and various cellular meta-bolic processes. Autism, according to this theory, is caused by external toxins—perhaps vaccines and also a range of other contaminants, such as viruses, industrial chemicals, and other such unnatural intrusions—that the affected person cannot effectively excrete. It is thus preventable, treatable, and potentially curable, and the first step is to get things out of the body that don't belong there—and keep them out.

At one such event I attended, the annual conference of the National Autism Association, the opening night's speaker reassured parents in the audience that their child's learning problems, misbehaviors, and un-controllable rages were not part of the child but instead came from the disease. The speaker was the chief executive officer of a clinic that had helped to sponsor the conference, one of a number of alternative medi-cal centers that strive to identify signs of contamination through various techniques, including laboratory testing for heavy metals in hair and urine samples, and then attempt to pull these pathogens out of children's bodies, using interventions that range from infrared saunas to chela-tion, a treatment for heavy metal poisoning. Many of these treatments are scientifically unproven and come with their own set of risks. But symptoms of physical distress can also be read as signs of progress, ways of making disorder newly visible in the body. "You ask: what did I do to your son?" the presenter said, describing parents' reactions to some of these manifestations—the rashes, the spikes in misbehavior, the lab tests that suddenly show problems where none were there before. "But it's a good thing—it means it's coming *out!*" Such a formulation offers hope in difficult moments. "When he is saying something violent, remember: it's not him or her. It's something else. There are biomedical roots. It's not the real him or her. And we treat it." The word *recover* is often used in these communities as a transitive verb: Parents recover their children *from* the autism that has taken them away. "Our goal" another speaker summarized, "is getting our children back. Pull them away from autism, and make them who they're meant to be."

A great deal of rhetorical work is done to depict autism as a bundle of unwanted elements that are separate from the child, who is assumed to have once existed (and anticipated to exist again in the future) with-out these impediments. A 2008 public service announcement from the National Autism Association, featuring an image of a huge sudsy bar of soap, started by announcing, "We're pretty good at cleaning up poop—it's the crap we can't handle." Examples of "crap" included not only "overly aggressive combination vaccine schedules that haven't been properly tested" but also

> continually being told our children's autism is a gift. Autism is not a gift. Our children are the gift. Autism is the inability to communicate, the inability to stay comfortable, the inability to stay safe. Autism is stomachaches and insomnia and seizures and head-banging and dozens of other symptoms unworthy of a bow. But our children are human beings worthy of prevention, treatment and hope for recovery.

Such rhetoric draws a clear separation between "our children" as human beings and the autism that afflicts them; the latter is defined as a laundry list of deficits and somatic discomforts. When I asked one parent how her 4-year-old son, now described as recovered and cheerfully sporting a National Autism Association T-shirt, made sense of this kind of material, she told me she wasn't sure. But she remembered that he once said to her: "I crumpled up autism and threw it in the garbage."

Although their emphasis on alternative medical practices and resistance to vaccination places such organizations well outside the medical mainstream, they are nonetheless politically influential: Representatives have sat on major government committees such as the Inter-Agency Autism Coordination Committee, responsible for determining directions and priorities for federally funded autism research in the United States, and this perspective has a powerful influence within Autism Speaks. Autism Speaks, in particular, is well known for rhetoric depicting autism as a malevolent force, antithetical to all that is good in life. One notorious advertisement from 2009 featured a cartoonishly villainous voice intoning things like "I am autism—I know where you live, and guess what? I live there, too. . . . I speak your language fluently—and with every voice I take away, I acquire yet another language. . . . I will fight to take away your hope—I will plot to rob you of your children and your dreams—I will make sure that every day you wake up you will cry . . ." and so on. A 2014 "Founders' Message" from founders Suzanne and Bob Wright ended with the highlighted words: "This disorder has taken our children away. It's time to get them back" (Wright & Wright, 2014).

The image of autism as a kidnapper is widespread; however, the metaphorical representation of psychiatric diagnostic entities as malevolent, child-stealing intruders isn't limited to autism. The "Ransom Notes" campaign of advertisements placed by the New York University (NYU) Child Study Center in 2007 depicted conditions such as autism alongside ADHD, bulimia, and depression as kidnappers holding kids for ransom (payment to be delivered, presumably, to the NYU Child Study Center). Enormous billboards taking the form of scrawled notes, some appearing handwritten and some made up of cutout letters, they said things like

> We are in possession of your son. We are making him squirm and fidget until he is a detriment to himself and those around him. Ignore this and your kid will pay.
> —ADHD

and

> We have taken your son. We have imprisoned him in a maze of darkness with no hope of ever getting out. Do nothing and see what happens.
> —Depression

alongside

> We have your son. We are destroying his ability for social interaction and driving him into a life of complete isolation. It's up to you now.
> —Asperger's Syndrome

The notes all ended with the warning: Don't let a psychiatric disorder take your child.

In recent years, the tide of public opinion has turned somewhat against these lurid, pathologizing representations. The "Ransom Notes" ads were taken down quickly—although not without initial resistance—after a public outcry. Autism Speaks has worked to soften its language since the passing of Suzanne Wright and some changing of the guard among its leadership, even going so far as to remove the word *cure* from its mission statement in 2016 (Diament, 2016). Defeat Autism Now!

changed its name to the Autism Research Institute, in response to requests from autistic people for whom the name felt like a "personal affront" (Edelson, n.d.).

However, the notion of psychiatric disorders as both separate from and antithetical to personhood continues to pervade clinical discourses, often in more subtle but still influential ways (see Luhrmann, 2000, and Weiner, 2011, for accounts). For example, the idea of a psychiatric condition as fundamentally separable from and incompatible with the full personhood of the affected person manifests in the common and widely accepted practice of "person-first language." Adopted from the disability advocacy community and recommended as a form of respectful communication around mental illnesses by numerous sources such as the American Psychological Association Style Guide, "person-first language" requires that one refer to disabilities separately from, and after, the person whom they affect: *Steve is a person with schizophrenia* rather than *Steve is schizophrenic* or *Steve is a schizophrenic*. "Labeling the person as the disability . . . dehumanizes the individual and equates the condition with the person" states one set of Guidelines for Reporting and Writing about People with Disabilities (Research and Training Center on Independent Living, 2008), urging writers to "put people first, not their disability" (p. 2). The idea behind person-first language is to honor the dignity and full personhood of the affected person. However, by positing that the way to do that is to depict the disability as separate from the person, this separation is further established as a necessary precondition of that personhood.

Like many autistic self-advocates, Lana is not on board with the assumptions of person-first language when it comes to autism. She explained:

> The whole notion of person-first language, to me, is almost like saying that it's a bad thing. Because you never say, like, *she has beauty. She has intelligence. We need to respect her person first and her beauty second.* No, you say, *she's beautiful. She's intelligent. She's creative*, you know. And those are all positive—and sometimes autism can be a positive: *she's autistic.* Whereas if you say, *she has a wart, she has cancer, she has allergies, she has autism,* it's kind of icky. Or sometimes you can just say like, *she's Italian. She's Jewish.* It's an identifying characteristic, but is just neutral. *She's autistic*: it's a fact. It's not a value statement.

However, her critique of person-first language does not apply to all her diagnoses:

> I have a million other diagnoses as well, and I don't think of those as part of me. I have Tourette's. I'd be very happy without it. It's just annoying. And it's not a part of me; it's something I *have*. And the same way, if I get depression, it's something I *have*. But autism—I don't think of it as something I have. I never say, *I have autism* or *I have Asperger's*. I prefer to say, *I am autistic*, because I'm autistic just like I am female. To me, being female isn't good or bad. It's just what I am, and I wouldn't change it. If I lived in another culture, another time, I probably would. But I think the same thing about autism.

Understanding the differentiation Lana draws here, between autistic as something that she *is* and depression as something that she *has*, requires understanding the divergent histories of the psychiatric traditions that produced each of these conditions in their current forms. Depression and Tourette's are diagnoses that emerged under an older paradigm of psychiatric diagnosis, one that delineates discrete disease entities consisting only of their negative manifestations. Being autistic, in the way that Lana is (which is, of course, quite different from what it would have meant to have that word applied to oneself in other historical moments), is a diagnostic status emerging out of a new approach to diagnosis, producing diagnostic entities that are not exclusively negative and that often feel inseparable from and in fact perhaps constitutive of the persons they affect. They delineate very different personal terrain.

The Main Thing Was That It Had to Make Sense

Psychiatric diagnostic categories as most Americans know them today are organized through the *Diagnostic and Statistical Manual of Mental Disorders*, or *DSM* for short—a manual published and intermittently updated by the American Psychiatric Association. A great deal of how we think about and act upon mental disorder—how patients understand their illness, how doctors treat their patients, how insurance companies reimburse doctors, how researchers develop treatments, how funding agencies allocate money to research—is shaped by the parameters of this system.

The *DSM* took on its current form in the late 1970s, during the revision from its second to third edition. Psychiatric diagnosis was in a crisis of reliability. The wide variation in approaches among practitioners was posing increasing problems for both the legitimacy of psychiatric diagnosis and its practical applications, just as the assessment and treatment of mental health problems was becoming an integral component of a growing array of federal and bureaucratic systems.[2] When Robert Spitzer took over as chairman of the DSM-III revision committee, he and his team were aiming, above all, to standardize diagnosis, providing an interdisciplinary common language to ensure that a psychoanalytically oriented psychiatrist in a Boston hospital would diagnose a given patient the same way as a behavior therapist in private practice in Arkansas. To do so, they designed checklists based on observable symptoms, under the assumption that these were likely to map onto underlying pathological processes. This categorical system—you meet criteria or you don't—provides the illusion of robustness around psychiatric categories: major depressive disorder is a real thing with sharp lines around it, something that a person either *has* or *does not have.*

In theory, these diagnoses were determined based on empirical data rather than etiological speculation; in practice, establishing these checklists of symptoms most often involved committees of experts forming a consensus around what symptoms intuitively seemed to go together. Journalist Alix Spiegel (2005), interviewing Spitzer for a *New Yorker* piece on the development of the *DSM-III* (American Psychiatric Association, 1980), asked him what criteria were used to decide whether to add a new mental disorder to the manual. His response was as follows:

> "How logical it was," he said, vaguely. "Whether it fit in. The main thing was that it had to make sense. It had to be logical." He went on, "For most of the categories, it was just the best thinking of people who seemed to have expertise in the area" (p. 59).

The result was a series of diagnoses that also functioned as common-sense folk categories, composed entirely of negative manifestations of a presumed but unseen underlying pathology. The correlations between symptoms that made a diagnostic category "make sense" were experiential, subjective, grounded in the self-report of a distressed patient.

Aspects of (for example) anxiety that were not easily observed by a clinician or reported by a patient were left out of the disease category: Causal factors such as repressed intrapsychic conflict or shifts in neurotransmitter uptake were excluded, as were potential benefits like the thrill of fear or the increased likelihood of avoiding dangerous circumstances. The *DSM-III* transformed wide swaths of human suffering and social deviance into discrete disease entities, sharply delineated and reified, exclusively negative in their impact, and located within but separable from the affected person, able to travel between patients and between contexts without changing in their fundamental nature. They functioned, in other words, like germs.

Medical historian Charles Rosenberg (2002) chronicles how *disease specificity*, "the notion that diseases can and should be thought of as entities existing outside the unique manifestations of illness in particular men and women" has become an increasingly prevalent organizing force in an "increasingly technical, specialized, and bureaucratized" (p. 237) context of care. Germ theory, the late 19th-century discovery that some diseases are caused by tiny, invisible entities traveling between bodies, became an organizing metaphor for these already developing trends in medical diagnosis. It made a "telling argument for the implicit assumption that disease could be understood as existing in some sense outside the body" and "communicated metaphorically the more abstract notion of disease entity as ideal type abstracted from its particular manifestations" (Rosenberg, 2007, 19). At the same time, it made "a powerful argument for a reductionist, mechanism-oriented way of thinking about the body and its felt malfunctions" (Rosenberg, 2002, p. 243).

However, in the case of the kinds of conditions that fall under the domain of psychiatric medicine, the hope that a clearer delineation of patterns of symptoms would lead to the discovery of corresponding underlying pathophysiological states was not realized. In an introduction to a series of articles describing upcoming changes to the diagnostic classification process, Darrel Regier (2007), the vice-chair of the task force planning the *DSM-5* (American Psychiatric Association, 2013), observed that the expectation that "highly specific phenomenological descriptions of disorders . . . would result in phenomenological subtypes that would eventually correlate with etiological and pathophysiological factors needed to validate these more precise clinical syndromes" has not been supported by the findings emerging out of genomics and neuroscience. "The pieces of this optimistic vision failed to fall neatly into place" (Regier, 2007, pp. S3–S4). By the end of the 20th century, a new paradigm was starting to emerge—one with very different implications for the relationship between self and disorder.

You Are Your Connectome

"Ever wonder what is it that makes you, you?" asks a 2012 Director's Blog post from National Institutes of Health (NIH) director Francis Collins, titled "The Symphony Inside Your Brain":

> These days some of the world's top neuroscientists might say: "You are your connectome." The connectome refers to the exquisitely interconnected network of neurons (nerve cells) in your brain. Like the genome, the microbiome, and other exciting "ome" fields, the effort to map the connectome and decipher the electrical signals that zap through it to generate your thoughts, feelings, and behaviors has become possible through development of powerful new tools and technologies. (para. 1)

The post introduces the Connectome Project, a massive, multisite NIH-funded initiative whose goal is to "map the brain's neural connections in their entirety" (para. 4). Previous efforts to understand the human brain, Collins explains in the post, focused on inferring the function of various individual brain regions—an approach he likens to

> listening to the string section (evaluating an isolated part of the brain) versus listening to an entire orchestra (the whole organ). If you listen only to the string or percussion section, you'll gain a pretty good understanding of how that particular group of instruments sounds. However, that experience would not compare to the experience of listening to the whole orchestra and chorus perform Beethoven's Symphony No. 9, the Ode to Joy. (para. 3)

The nature and beauty of the symphonic self are not found in individual pieces but emerge from the connections that make up the whole, a network that "generate[s] your thoughts, feelings, and behaviors" (Collins,

2012, para. 1). The term *connectome* evokes connotations of systematic completeness, "inspired by earlier projects that mapped the complete structure of entities in a particular biological domain—most notably the Human Genome Project" (Haueis & Slaby, 2017)—an approach that also characterizes such large-scale initiatives as the NIMH BRAIN (Brain Research through Advancing Innovative Neurotechnologies) initiative.

The organizing metaphors of such projects foreground systems of connection over discrete locations. Metaphors of "wiring" and "circuitry" are pervasive within this approach to psychiatric diagnosis. The advent of brain imaging, as anthropologist of science Joseph Dumit (2004) has observed, produced a ubiquitous image of the brain as a series of blazing regions, areas of relative activation or inactivity providing clues about the depression or schizophrenia supposedly located within. Now, those rainbow patches are increasingly looking old-fashioned, and articles about the Big New Brain Science are accompanied instead by images of the brain made up of wiry bundles of rainbow filaments, cables, and connectors. In a 2010 article in *Scientific American*, titled "Faulty Circuits," Tom Insel, then the director of the National Institute of Mental Health, announced that, thanks to new neuroimaging technologies, "mental disorders can, for the first time, be studied as abnormalities in the connections between distant areas of the brain. . . . Brain regions that function together to carry out normal mental operations can be thought of as analogous to electrical circuits. And the latest research shows that the malfunctioning of entire circuits may underlie many mental disorders" (p. 44). The language of brain circuitry evokes the image of the brain as a sophisticated electronic computing machine, conjuring associations of both a robust objectivity and a vulnerability to "faults" that originate from within.

The goal of the Human Connectome Project, and others like it, is thus not only to celebrate and better appreciate "what makes you, you" but also to identify and eliminate certain aspects of that system: the conditions identified as "neurological disorders." "With a detailed connectome map of a normal human brain," Collins (2012) goes on to say,

> I believe we will gain a better understanding of the roots of human neurological disorders, including schizophrenia, autism spectrum disorders, and other baffling conditions that may arise from abnormal "wiring" dur-

ing brain development. This knowledge should yield new and better ways to detect, treat, and, ultimately, prevent the brain disorders that currently disrupt and devastate so many lives. (para. 6)

In the shift from what Collins refers to metaphorically as "listening to the string section" (looking for discrete disease entities limited to particular locations: a pathogen model of illness) to "listening to the whole orchestra and chorus" (attending to a rich network of connections out of which phenomena are emergent), a new kind of clinical entity is produced—one that is produced from within, rather than from without, a system that is interconnected, not location-specific. The stakes of detection and elimination are thus significantly different, to an extent that is undertheorized in newly developing diagnostic systems.

Disease States Heretofore Unrecognized

In 1999, representatives from the NIMH and the American Psychiatric Association convened a meeting, the purpose of which was to lay the groundwork for the next revision of the *DSM*. Much like the revision from *DSM-II* (American Psychiatric Association, 1968) to *DSM-III* (American Psychiatric Association, 1980), this revision was seen as an opportunity for a comprehensive overhaul in the basic assumptions around which the classification system itself was designed, addressing pervasive dissatisfactions with the current system. This time around, the concerns lay less with the reliability than the validity of diagnostic categories. The *DSM-III* and *DSM-IV* (American Psychiatric Association, 1994) had established a common language for diagnosis (although consistency around the application of diagnostic labels was still not where the architects of the system had hoped)—but questions remained as to whether that language referred to anything robustly real. Both researchers and clinical practitioners were finding significant overlap between categories—patients who experienced both anxiety and depression or mood states that seemed like a combination of both. Nor did the sharp divisions between the sick and the well, implied by a categorical system, hold up in research and practice. Psychopharmaceutical medications that had once been lauded for their ability to specifically target particular disorders were instead being applied across a wide range of conditions—"antipsychotics" used for treatment-resistant depression and other mood disorders, "antidepressants" that found their largest markets in social anxiety—with limited overall efficacy in each case. These concerns motivated attempts toward a comprehensive overhaul in the basic structure of psychiatric diagnosis.

These attempts were premised on a return to a focus on physiological cause over subjective symptom descriptions and their consensus interpretation: etiology over phenomenology. In a series of white papers produced in 2002 to guide the revision, titled "A Research Agenda for DSM-V," one set of authors observed that this shift

> would represent a highly laudable achievement for psychiatry and would help move the specialty into the mainstream of modern medicine, where etiology and pathophysiology have replaced descriptive symptomatology as the fundamental basis for making diagnostic distinctions. (Charney et al., 2002, p. 33)

The white papers covered a wide range of topics but converged on a primary set of recommendations: a diagnostic system that was based on neurobiological etiology drawing on cutting-edge science rather than on subjective symptom report; that was organized around continuous spectrums rather than dichotomous, you're-in-or-you're out categories; and whose aim was presymptomatic prevention, as well as treatment, of the newly identified diagnostic entities. Its architects looked forward to a future in which

> it will be discovered that specific combinations of genes will relate to constellations of abnormalities in many brain-based functions—including but not limited to the regulation of mood, anxiety, perception, learning, memory, aggression, eating, sleeping, and sexual function—that will coalesce to form disease states heretofore unrecognized. (Charney et al., p. 70)

Unlike the current system, contours of these new disease states would not be determined by subjective judgments about what "made sense" as a diagnostic category. Instead, their form would "coalesce" through the seemingly objective tracing of patterns of physiologically grounded relationships between elements: combinations of genes associated with constellations of observed abnormalities in basic brain functions.

Subjective experiences of impairment, and the associated value judgments about what kinds of experiences belong or do not belong in a clinical category, have less of a place in such an objectively determined system. In another of these white papers, Lehman, Alexopoulos, Goldman, Feste, and Ünstün (2002) observe that achieving a categorization system "driven by knowledge about etiology and risk factors rather than by phenomenology" (p. 203) will require us to take a step back from considering subjective matters such as distress or disability to be necessary elements of disorders. Within such a framework,

> the presence or absence of distress or disability should not govern the determination of the presence of a mental disorder or the need for treatment; removing the requirement for impairment from diagnostic criteria will encourage early intervention for those at risk for future morbidity and death rather than delaying intervention until after significant morbidity has occurred. (Lehman et al., 2002, pp. 203–204)

Presymptomatic identification and the prevention of disease states are prioritized over what is sometimes referred to as "palliative" management of distressing symptoms, while subjective experiences and judgments of impairment are removed from the delineation of disease states. There are two intertwined consequences to this move. On one hand, multivalent syndromes are produced. If the contents of disease categories are not limited to observable manifestations that clinical consensus agrees are problematic and are based instead on neurobiological substrates, there is no reason to believe that problematic elements are all they will contain. On the other hand, the goal is to intervene on these syndromes before their complexities manifest, allowing them to continue being represented as exclusively negative disease states.

When the time came to produce the new manual, the architects of the new system faced the same problem that confronted their predecessors: there was not yet enough research data to support the new system. Much of the existing research that was being done was organized around *DSM* categories, thus making it difficult to use that data to deconstruct those categories and create something new. When it was released in 2013 by the American Psychiatric Association, the *DSM-5* was formally similar in many ways to previous editions, organized around symptom checklists and categorical diagnoses. There were a few significant changes: The "multiaxial system" that had separated mental disorders and developmental disabilities along separate axes in previous editions was eliminated, emphasizing the commonalities between these conditions over their differences. And the five different categories of "pervasive developmental disorder"—including autistic disorder, Asperger's syndrome, and PDD-NOS (pervasive developmental disorder, not otherwise specified)—were rolled into a single category of "autism spectrum disorder," with a specifier for level of severity defined by the extent of the person's need for support, thus formalizing autism's place as a forerunner of these transformed diagnostic entities.

At the same time as the *DSM* revision process was beginning to run up against the limitations of data that had been developed using *DSM* categories, however, a new initiative was launched through the NIMH, with the goal of spurring research that was not limited by these existing categories but could instead support a new diagnostic system. In a somewhat incendiary "Director's Blog" post written shortly before the release of the long-awaited new *DSM*, Tom Insel, then the director of the NIMH, spelled out the ways in which the newly launched Research Domain Criteria Project (RDoC) would address the many flaws still troubling the *DSM*. Rather than focusing on symptoms, he argued, "we need to begin collecting the genetic, imaging, physiologic, and cognitive data to see how all the data—not just the symptoms—cluster" (Insel, 2013, para. 4). RDoC picks up where *A Research Agenda for DSM-V* left off, identifying clusters of neurobiological phenomena across levels of analysis to break free from existing subjective categories and symptoms. Its goal is to produce an etiologically grounded system that can support the presymptomatic detection and prevention of mental illnesses, which have been reconceptualized as innate neurodevelopmental trajectories.

The new system would be dimensional, rather than categorical, following the NIMH's Strategic Plan for RDoC, which committed to studying "the full range of variation, from normal to abnormal" along these dimensions (Cuthbert, 2014). The dimensions around which RDoC is organized—"negative valence systems," such as threat and loss; "positive valence systems," such as approach motivation; "cognitive systems," such as attention, perception, and memory; and "social processes," such as affiliation and attachment—are not lists of troubling symptoms but instead constitute many of the most fundamental and consequential ways we engage with the world around us. Its purview spans not only how we suffer but also how we desire, learn, attend, and remember; how we perceive ourselves and others; how we grieve our losses; how we bond with those we love.

While the *DSM-5* (American Psychiatric Association, 2013) and its categorical disease entities would continue to organize clinical practice, RDoC was intended as a guide to funding priorities for research. The result has been a widening of the conceptual divide between basic science research and clinical practice in psychiatry. While treatment interventions are still being guided by a conception of particular disorders as discrete disease entities, separable from the affected person and limited to their unwanted manifestations, clinical research structures are delineating an entity with different contours, not limited to impairment and more focused on fundamental human capacities deeply intertwined with surrounding meaning-worlds. Such approaches produce diagnostic entities that are more package-like than pathogen-like—and that thus feel closer to a description of not merely what we suffer from but also who we are.

A Different Pattern of Processing That Can Bring Tremendous Strengths

Conditions once defined as sets of impairments are increasingly being reconceptualized as comprehensive forms of neurogenetic organization, and as they do, they are increasingly recognized to involve a wide range of attributes. For example, while dyslexia has traditionally been defined as a learning disability that produces difficulty in reading, a recent spate of research takes dyslexia instead as a brain-wide difference in information processing patterns; looking at it this way reveals advantages, in some contexts, as well as difficulties in others. A 2012 book called *The Dyslexic Advantage: Unlocking the Potential of the Dyslexic Brain* (Eide & Eide, 2012) identifies four different kinds of strengths "linked to particular cognitive and structural brain features common in individuals with dyslexia" (Eide & Eide, 2012 p. 2). In an interview with *WIRED* magazine

(Venton, 2011), these authors critiqued the "big misconception . . . that dyslexia is fundamentally a learning disorder which is accompanied only by problems, rather than a different pattern of processing that can bring tremendous strengths in addition to the well-known challenges" (para. 8). Instead, they argue that people who receive the diagnosis of dyslexia have a comprehensive difference in the overall organization of their brains, predisposing them to a processing style that helps them perceive big-picture relationships and narrative connections—thus explaining findings by business school professor Julie Logan that there are high levels of dyslexia among entrepreneurs (Logan, 2009). "It's not a book about something these individuals *have*," the authors assure us in its Introduction. "It's a book about who they *are*" (Eide & Eide, 2012, p. 1). Similarly, in a *New York Times* op-ed titled "Defining My Dyslexia," dyslexic author Blake Charlton (2013) argued that, while dyslexia has brought him significant challenges, "scientific evidence and social observation will continue to show that defining dyslexia based solely on its weaknesses is inaccurate and unjust" (para. 3). As the lens through which we view dyslexia widens through a big-picture view of whole-brain organizational patterns, the phenomena that emerge are no longer limited to functional impairments. Instead, they expand to include phenomena such as entrepreneurship (and, as in Charlton's case, a knack for creative writing—he's written a series of fantasy novels featuring a young wizard cursed to misspell his spells).

The multivalence of syndromes defined through neurogenetic correlations, manifesting both within individuals and through patterns of family heritability, is particularly striking in the case of autism, in which impairments and strengths correlate in complex ways that suggest that they may be part of the same physiological syndrome. In a population-based survey of 8-year-old twins, for example, Vital, Ronald, Wallace, and Happé (2009) found that even among those with no spectrum diagnosis, children with unusual abilities showed significantly more traits related to autism spectrum conditions than those without such abilities. Examining the degree of correlation between identical and fraternal twins suggested that the association between these traits and special skills was, in large part, due to shared genetic effects. "Put simplistically," stated a later article reviewing these findings, "some genetic factors that predispose to ASC [autism spectrum condition]-like traits (and specifically RRBIs [restricted or repetitive behaviors/interests]) also predispose to talent" (p. 1372).

However, these manifestations, outside the traditional purview of medical practice, are frequently missed by a clinical gaze focused only on problems. Furthermore, the differences that are observed are often interpreted through a pathologizing lens. In a 2006 commentary in the journal *Behavioral and Brain Sciences*, autism scientists Morton Anne Gernsbacher, Michelle Dawson, and Laurent Mottron demonstrate that while the "empirical literature is replete with demonstrations of autistics' superiority in numerous perceptual, reasoning, and comprehension tasks . . . each of these statistically significant demonstrations of autistic superiority is labeled by its authors as a harmful dysfunction" (p. 2; see also Dawson & Mottron, 2009). Superior performance on block design tasks is interpreted as a manifestation of weak central coherence; superior recognition memory is attributed to misapplication of attention to shallow features of stimuli; superior ability to ignore misleading context features is given as evidence of deficits in perception. The complex, multivalent phenomena produced through the neurodevelopmental turn get carved down into partial pictures characterized only by impairment.

Very, Very Targeted Biological Treatments

This focus on impairment is maintained through situating research on neurodevelopmental conditions within clinical settings that are organized around the investigation and remediation of problems. NIMH-funded research, for all it supposedly now aims to delineate the full spectrum of human functioning, does not tend to recruit participants in business schools where Julie Logan found her dyslexic entrepreneurs or at the universities where the broader autism phenotype is producing single-minded scientists or at the protests where Kieran's incandescent anger gets put to a purpose. In a 2014 discussion of how research studies under RDoC would recruit a wider range of participants to understand the full range of a phenomenon along a particular dimension, RDoC Unit Director Bruce Cuthbert suggests that

> samples for a study of reward circuit activity (as relevant to anhedonia and/or mania) might be drawn from virtually the entire population of

treatment-seeking adults—mood/anxiety spectrum, psychotic spectrum, eating disorders, personality disorders; for appropriate exploration of dimensionality, the sample would also include relatively minor psycho-pathology such as an adjustment reaction diagnosis as well as those in-dividuals who do not meet criteria for any diagnosis. A similar approach might be used to study executive function in children across a range of autism spectrum, attention-deficit/hyperactivity disorder, and mood/anxiety disorders (and once again, those who do not meet criteria for any disorder). (p. 32, emphasis added)

Note the parentheses. Although the need to include some participants who are not presenting with clinically significant distress is briefly acknowledged, the focus is on recruiting participants through clini-cal settings that aggregate those who are suffering and foreground that suffering over other elements of experience. This approach produces a distorted image of a condition, in which its problematic parts stand in for the entirety of the whole.

While I was in Park City, I spent some time at a lab that was con-ducting neuroimaging studies and clinical trials of pharmaceutical treatments for autism. "How would you define an autism spectrum dis-order to someone who'd never heard of it?" I asked the lead scientist, Dr. Clarkson, at the start of our interview.

"I describe autism as characterized by three core symptom domains: social impairments, language impairments, and behavior impairments," he began and then gave some examples about what each of those im-pairments could be. This is a definition of autism as a disease entity: characterized by an observable pattern of problematic symptoms. Yet the autism that the clinic sought to identify and intervene on was a dif-ferent autism: a presymptomatic profile of molecular and physiological states. When I asked him to describe the overarching goal of the center, he replied:

What we're doing is, from a whole multitude of angles, looking at kind
of the basic science elements of autism, trying to identify what the
susceptibility genes are, what's the etiology, trying to unravel es-
sentially what the biological cause of autism is. That's certainly one of
our core missions. Then what we're trying to do is take what we learn

there to developing treatment—because, in the end, that's really what people need. That is the driving force behind this.

ELIZABETH: If you were to have success with that mission and come to a greater understanding of the biological etiology of autism spectrum disorders, what do you think would change in the world, or in the lives of people with autism?

DR. CLARKSON: I think there would be the option for prevention, first of all. If you could pick it up in utero, it would be nice if people had the choice much like they have with Fragile X or Down's syndrome. Or alternatively, with that choice, if you knew exactly what on like a cellular level some of the core deficits are, you could develop very, very targeted biological treatments. So that on sort of both ends of the spectrum you'd have an array of options that could really manage this disease, and people with autism could probably function significantly better.

In *Tracing Autism: Uncertainty, Ambiguity, and the Affective Labor of Neuroscience* (2017), Des Fitzgerald describes a passionate and caring group of neuroscientists, deeply motivated to help their intriguing patients. But they struggle with a fundamental uncertainty: the condition on which they seek to intervene consistently eludes their efforts to locate it in the body. Aware of the ambiguous status of autism, they nonetheless strive to articulate it as a particular kind of thing on which they could act in a familiar way, to reduce or remove. The scientists I got to know in Park City were similarly motivated by a strong desire to help the people that they saw every day, who were struggling with extraordinarily difficult issues. "I think everybody who works here has this very sincere and kind of passionate interest in autism," Dr. Clarkson told me when I asked him what was the most important thing for me to know about the work of the research center.

Most of the people that you've been interacting with are clinical researchers, so they're not just interested in asking intellectual research questions. They're actually interested in working with children. I think they get a lot of satisfaction by seeing kids improve and by having a real impact. . . . It's kind of a wonderful place in that sense: because we're all working towards what we think is this greater good, in the hope that we can achieve success as a center, achieve success personally, and we can help other people to achieve success in their daily lives.

The view of autism held by Dr. Clarkson and his colleagues, in which autism is represented by its most problematic manifestations, makes a great deal of sense, given the stories that he and his colleagues hear, day after day, as they interview families who are at their wits' end about the problems that trouble them, looking at whether the treatments they test have led to any measurable improvement in symptoms. Yet the areas on which this work aims to intervene—susceptibility genes, mechanisms of action—may be producing not only the impairments associated with autism that show up in these interactions but its whole, complex picture.

Meanwhile, the rolling-together of a wide variety of life experiences into a single *autism spectrum* supports attention to their common problems over their multivalent variations in manifestation. I asked Dr. Clarkson what kind of approaches might make the most sense for people in the range of autism often referred to as "high-functioning." "The same thing, actually," he replied. He described some of the ways that people with Asperger's and related conditions still struggle—the anxiety, depression, and alienation, the risk of humiliation when carefully crafted coping mechanisms fail. "If the core of the disorder is manifesting but at sort of a less significant level, you can still extrapolate and assume that the same neurochemical systems are involved, just perhaps to a lesser extent. But you can still intervene with the same regulatory agents."

But the distinction between autism—the disease on which they aim to intervene with regulatory agents—and other phenomena—such as the capacity for intense fascination and persistence—is not so easy to draw. One of the scientists I interviewed there was very involved in training graduate students in the diagnostic assessments used to determine whether potential participants met inclusion criteria for research studies. She told me about the challenge of teaching trainees to distinguish diagnostically between a 14-year-old who will stop talking about bugs when they see their interlocutor isn't interested and a 14-year-old who keeps talking about it anyway. "One area that we're not very good at is the difference between [people with Asperger's and] these really gifted kids that have a lot to share, that don't have a lot of opportunity to share it, that may or may not be Asperger's," she observed. "Like, we don't know what to do with those kids in general, so it's hard to tell the trainees what to do with those kids."

The scientists in the Park City lab knew that they were facing tricky philosophical questions about the distinction between abnormality and pathology—where to classify the failure to stop talking about something that the person you're talking to doesn't want to hear? "Where are we drawing the line between someone who's just an odd person and someone who we're giving this label as having Asperger's disorder or being on the spectrum?" another scientist on the team mused to me. Standardized tests and clinical diagnostic measures "are helpful in drawing the line. But yeah, we're sort of being asked to draw a line between pathology and just being weird." He struggled with this expectation. "It's not easy to do."

We Will Know Where the Enemy Is

In 2001, psychiatrist Nancy Andreasen's popular book *Brave New Brain: Conquering Mental Illness in the Era of the Genome* heralded "an era when two large knowledge bases will meet and mingle: the map of the human genome and the map of the human brain" (Andreasen, 2001, p. 318). After a series of chapters describing lives torn apart by disorders such as major depressive disorder and schizophrenia, the concluding section, titled "Defining the Target: Using Guidance from Maps of Brain Terrain," gives us an optimistic progress update on "the war against mental illness." Andreasen tells readers that

> recent decades have not only added many weapons to our arsenal for attack on mental illnesses, but they have also given us a map of the terrain on many different levels in the cascade from genes through brain and mind. We no longer need to aim blindly and hope we might hit the enemy. . . . During the next several decades, we can expect to identify the abnormalities in brain geography and topography that define the various types of mental illnesses. Once this is accomplished, we will know where the enemy is. The techniques of molecular biology will give us the capacity to do precision bombing, while our maps of brain terrain will give us the targets at which to aim. (pp. 319–320)

This is a performance of the "Ode to Joy" in which the principal violinist plays some sour notes and gets taken out by a drone strike. The coexistence of pathogen-based logics of elimination and whole-package mapping of the self-as-terrain produce a macabre depiction of self-inflicted harm, in which the map and the target are conflated.

The kinds of linguistic slippage posed by divided medicalization, in which one kind of autism (autism as a pathogen) comes to represent another (autism as a whole package), presents a particular kind of risk. When conditions such as autism are targeted for intervention and change as if they consisted only of their unwanted attributes, we risk suppressing a wider range of human qualities *despite*—and, ironically, in many ways *because of*—medical infrastructures that deliberately exclude such attributes from their domain of intervention. In the next chapter, we will see this process unfold in action, guided by logics of extrusion that guard both bodies and clinic boundaries. Paradoxically, in the attempt to keep such nonpathological elements as creativity, talent, and pleasure outside of the purview of medical intervention, these characteristics become invisible in a way that makes them vulnerable.

It has always been true that some people develop dramatically differently from how their society expects, resulting in profound and pervasive difficulties managing developmental tasks and fulfilling social roles. In recent years, through the expansion of the autism spectrum, these difficulties have become the grounds for an ongoing referendum on sociality itself, one that has come to revolve around issues of flexibility, spontaneity, and the integration of overabundant stimuli. Autism spectrum disorder diagnoses, and the various social assemblages that spring up around them, bring together a very diverse group of people who share at least some of a broad pool of attributes—social struggles, rigidity or repetition or hyper-focus, a fraught relationship with sensation—rendering those attributes particularly salient above others. Other characteristics that tend to travel along with those particular manifestations (ranging from problems with organization and planning to a deep appreciation for the kind of external systems that can assist with those processes) get aggregated as well, without being explicitly articulated as part of the category. By bringing together and rendering explicit the connections between some continuous aspects (impairment, isolation) while underemphasizing others (aesthetics, patterns of affiliation), the diagnostic category takes characteristics that might, in many cases, do complex cultural work (rigidity, a desire for repetition and consistency, a decentralizing of dyadic social reciprocity, a focus on stable local connections over fluid global gestalts) and strengthens their conceptual association with the notion of biologically determined functional impairment—thus opening them up to biological preventative intervention.

In a pair of sensitive and nuanced explorations of the attitudes of autism scientists toward their work, both Silverman (2012) and Fitzgerald (2017) have addressed the ethics and implications of neuroscientific practice by demonstrating that practitioners bring a critical ethical sensibility to their work. What this line of reasoning leaves out is the broader network within which these practitioners' work takes place, within which intentions in one direction may power movements toward different ends. As Pellicano and Stears (2011) have observed, claims to neutrality or other specific stances on the part of autism researchers do not restrict or define the uses to which that research can be put.

The neurodevelopmental turn and its associated logic of plasticity are characterized by an attention to our fundamental openness to the environment and our capacity to change over time as we are shaped by our interactions with that environment. These paradigms unearth conditions that are multivalent, identitarian, and worlded. As such, they offer an invitation to cultivate a clinical science that is more in touch with the meaningful worlds we inhabit and transform. But many clinical infrastructures are ill equipped to accommodate these transformative possibilities. As a result, we instead see a collapse of those evoked worlds onto the individual embodied person. When physiological characteristics, contained within selves as closed systems, become an explanation for lifeworlds in such a way as to systematically occlude broader social, cultural, and environmental forces and factors, it instead contributes to the attenuation of social bonds. In the process, that which we cherish becomes the target of intervention that feels like violence. The potential for such intervention poses a deep threat to people like Lana, for whom autism is a constitutive and intimate element of identity—and perhaps also to those of us who want to live in a world characterized by a rich diversity of approaches to that world, who may have reason to fear that the war against mental illness is now being waged against the symphony of the self.

6

The Division of a Syndrome

Guess What I Did with the Doctor Today?

I am sitting in a room full of psychologists, neuropsychologists, and psychology trainees: the staff of the Asperger Center. The center is a clinic located within the psychiatry department of the Hayes School of Medicine, a large urban medical school in Park City, a city a few hours away from Brookfield. It recently received a sizable private donation to establish programs devoted to the needs of children, adolescents, and young adults with Asperger's syndrome. The center is heavily advertised and occupies a suite of shiny new rooms in a downtown office building, adorned with the glowing logo of the Department of Psychiatry. The program is led by Dr. Martina Grace; with 15 years of experience working with people with Asperger's, she is generally considered one of the experts in the field.

We in this room call ourselves the Group Group. Although the Asperger Center staff do some individual, one-on-one work with their patients, the majority of the staff's work consists of putting together groups. Their goal is to provide opportunities for the center's patients, many of whom have few friends, few chances to interact with peers, and little idea what to do with the chances they do have, to spend time together in a way that will give them some practice interacting with other people in a way that feels good rather than awful. Simply putting them in a room together and letting them get to socializing won't do it; if that kind of unstructured interaction worked for them, they would have made friends on the playground or in the classroom already. Instead, the groups place young people with Asperger's into interactions structured around a common interest: history, sports, theater, bugs.

Once it became clear that an ethnographic researcher would not be a good fit at the newly reorganized program I had initially arranged to observe at the Hayes Center, Dr. Grace had invited me into the Group Group. (Its members seemed a bit more comfortable with weirdo outsiders than the rest of the medical school). Intrigued by my anthropological project and reassured by my clinical training, she figured the best way for me to understand the culture of the Group Group would be to help lead a group myself. So I work with a graduate student in psychology and a drama teacher to run an improvisational theater group for 6- to 9-year-old kids with Asperger's. Once a week I accompany the Exploring the City Group for college students with Asperger's, led by James, a behavior therapist, and Wendy, the administrative coordinator of the center, as we bowl at a local bowling alley or navigate the Aquarium on a crowded Saturday afternoon. The Group Group also runs a History Discussion Group and a Sports Talk Group and has a slew of other programs constantly under development: filmmaking, a chess club, a group where the kids work together on building a robot. It's an unusual set of pursuits for a group of mental health professionals; I know from my own clinical psychology training that psychologists aren't usually taught how to bowl or analyze baseball scores in graduate school. The work took us out of our professional comfort zone on a regular basis.

For example, today Wendy has suggested that the young adults of the Exploring the City Group go play Skee-Ball. Wendy is from the Midwest, where Skee-Ball is apparently a big thing, and she misses it. She thinks the people in the group might like to play Skee-Ball, too, and we're running out of local tourist destinations to explore. The problem is, in the city we're in, all the Skee-Ball arcades are in bars. Could we take our patients to a bar?

"Well, I mean, I wouldn't take them to a *bar*," Ellen the postdoc says matter-of-factly. She is just finishing up her training and very, very professional, in pearls and a navy blazer.

"What if it was during the day, though?" Wendy mused.

"Still . . ." Ellen is unconvinced.

"I mean, we would take them to a restaurant," James the behavior therapist points out. "They serve alcohol in restaurants."

Ellen shakes her head ruefully, resigned, laughing. *"Guess what I did with the doctor today?"* she quips, in mimicry of an imagined patient. The room dissolves into laughter with her.

I heard this laughter a lot at the Asperger Center. It was a particular kind of laughter, pealing out in sudden, shared bursts, just following a brief pause as we all glanced at each other around the room. The laughter—sometimes delighted, sometimes anxious, often both at once—was an acknowledgment that we were doing a very strange kind of medicine. As Luhrmann (2000) points out in her description of the "foxhole hilarity" of psychiatrists managing the contradictory imperatives of contemporary mental health care, laughter is a way to manage contradictions, acknowledge paradoxes, and cope with seemingly impossible demands. At the Asperger Center, laughter signaled moments when the roles and responsibilities of these health care providers were shifting in unexpected directions; it acknowledged discrepancies between their expectations and their reality. Such laughter indexed the paradox that the Group Group faced: They were working at a medical center to treat a medical condition, but the best ways to treat it didn't feel very medical at all.

The neurodevelopmental turn and its expansion of psychiatric practice into wider and wider arenas of social life, captured in the nascent diagnosis of Asperger's syndrome, was changing not only the way people diagnosed with this condition viewed themselves but also the way medical providers viewed themselves and their role. When did teaching teenagers how to make friends become a medical intervention? How did the therapeutic space occupied by the clinic come to include the bowling alley, the Aquarium, crowded buses, and the dirty, twisting streets of downtown? What kind of doctor takes her patients to bars? *Who are we, and what are we doing here?* As medical categorizations and classifications expanded beyond the borders of the body to examine and remedy disorders of social life in the world, the changing demands and imperatives of that work brought about shifts in the practice of practitioners. As Asperger's became medicalized, medicine was becoming Aspergerized—characterized by an attention to the interaction between the person and their world, giving rise to interventions that are playful and social, determined by pleasures as well as pathologies, driven by the goal of expanding relationships rather than containing contagion.

However, this process of change met with a great deal of resistance, both implicit and explicit, from the existing infrastructures and practices of a medical institution accustomed to a particular model of illness and associated treatment practices. The policies and practices of the medical center were designed to manage, control, and eliminate diseases: damaging, discrete, and often objectively measurable phenomena contained within individual bodies. The Asperger Center clinicians, on the other hand, saw Asperger's syndrome in a different way: as a package of characteristics, traveling together as a neurogenetically interconnected system, manifesting at the interface between the person and their world, with effects that could be positive, negative, neutral, or all of the above. Working effectively to remedy the troubles caused by Asperger's, according to this model, called for interventions that were aesthetic, interactive, and often pleasurable. These interventions crossed and complicated the clinic's carefully maintained boundaries, between the inside and the outside of both the building and the body. The two models of disorder and their associated practices did not easily coexist but instead came into frequent conflict. In the end, the elements of Asperger's syndrome that least fit within the existing medical paradigm were not successfully incorporated into that paradigm but instead came to be selectively excluded from it. What remained was a version of a condition that shared a name with its more expansively conceived counterpart, while lacking many of its valued and vital elements.

Deeply shaped by heuristics, assumptions, and practices that organize psychiatric diagnosis around the identification and elimination of discrete disease entities, the work of medicine as codified in the psychiatric clinic is not well prepared to accommodate the new diagnostic entities of the neurodevelopmental turn. Symptoms, meanings, and treatment practices that cannot fit an entrenched "pathogen model" of illness are gradually moved outside of the psychiatric clinic, into educational, recreational, or subcultural arenas; the medical version of the condition that remains is lacking critical pieces. This is the end point of the process I call *divided medicalization*. A condition whose contours are delineated through one set of medical rubrics and practices is then refracted through another. The result is a situation in which two slightly but significantly different concepts share the same name. And the clinic, whose healing work motivates much of the research organized around these diagnostic entities, is left holding a medical model of the condition divested of its pleasures, creations, and collaborations: a shadow of its former self.

Having Fun in the Therapeutic World

I spend much of my time at the center drawing things on large pieces of poster board. I'm not very good at drawing, but it turns out I'm better at it than either Susan or Anna, the two other Drama Group leaders. And the Drama Group needs a lot of things drawn on poster board: daily schedules, illustrated diagrams of Good Audience Position (*CLOSE your mouth! LOOK with your eyes! LISTEN with your ears! SIT on your seat!*), scenery and backdrops, a bridge for the troll in our production of *The Three Billy Goats Gruff.*

These visual supports, points of unambiguous, shared reference that scaffold our interactions, are critical for keeping the group oriented and organized. Most of the kids in the group don't even seem to know where their bodies are most of the time—they run around wildly, crashing into one another and the walls, or else they hold very, very, very still, assessing the situation as thoroughly as possible before moving a muscle. So we make a big circle on the floor with masking tape. It serves as an impromptu delineation of the audience from the stage, and it helps us all figure out who we are and what we're supposed to be doing at any given moment. We also use a lot of props and costumes to signal shifts between roles and their associated expectations. When you're in the wolf suit, you can growl and roar as much as you like; when you're out of the wolf suit, try to rein it in.

The Drama Group, in addition to its three leaders, has four members: two little girls and two little boys, all between the ages of 6 and 9. We usually spend the first 10 or 15 minutes getting everybody to sit on the tape circle and roll a ball from one person to the next, making eye contact and saying something nice to the person they're rolling the ball to. "That's a nice shirt, Rachel!" says Angela, passing her the ball. Rachel catches it, whispers something inaudible, and passes the ball to Jeriah. "Do you know the Mitzvah Man, the Mitzvah Man, the Mitzvah Man?" Jeriah sings. He is obsessed with taking old-fashioned popular songs (in this case, it's "Do You Know the Muffin Man?") and giving them lyrics about Judaism. He also likes to give people funny names. "Here you go, Mr. Wiggles!" He passes the ball to Juan. Juan throws the ball at the window.

We can't work on Pass the Ball for too long because we have a number of items on our schedule, and if we go off the schedule, the kids start to get agitated. The schedule, much like the circle, is our anchor in a world where nothing stays still. It's up on the wall, drawn every day in big letters on a big piece of poster board, and we can always direct attention to it when things get confusing. "Jeriah, is it time to sing a song? What does it say on the schedule? It says: AUDIENCE PRACTICE!" Audience Practice is when we sit on the tape circle and practice Good Audience Position, a key element of which is not singing songs while other people are performing. The kids take turns stepping into the circle and practice acting out roles they may also play in life: teacher and student, shop clerk and customer, parent and child. In later workshops, we add things like Costume Practice and Pretending With Props.

The workshop is an hour long, and by the time it's over each week, everyone is exhausted. If we run a moment past the scheduled end time, the room quickly fills with a diffuse existential panic about whether parents will still be in the waiting room, whether the dog will still get fed, whether the world will still be there when we finally get done. We end each week by singing a song all together about how it's "Time to Say Good-bye." Jeriah always wants to sing "It's Time to Say *Shalom*" instead; by the end of the 6-week workshop, it's caught on, and everyone is singing it that way.

"I don't know whether the psychiatry department appreciated what went on in that room," Anna told me when I interviewed her sometime later about her experiences running the drama program at the Asperger Center. During the time we had worked together, she had frequently described a sense of conflict between what she once described as the "clinician culture and the actor culture." She felt a pervasive sense of discomfort on the part of the psychiatry staff toward her attempts to integrate artistic work into medical practice, even though that's what she had gotten hired specifically to do. "I get the impression that [the Drama Group] was a little too out there for them. That it was not something that they were going to allow to happen again." Although an artistic approach to Asperger's was initially embraced by the medical center, Anna found that in the end, the tensions were too great for the program to be maintained:

> It's called a *play* for a reason. And that sense of freedom, and having the opportunity to have incredible things being created, it sometimes has a certain kind of behavior that is a little too free-spirited. In a therapeutic

[setting], it's not behavior that can be tolerated, and I felt that. It wasn't something that I wanted to change because I couldn't, but I recognized that making noise, and even in art, making a mess was not something that could happen. Having fun wasn't [something that could happen] in the therapeutic world.

Having fun, or at least creating situations in which other people had fun, was, in fact, a central goal of many of the Group Group's interventions. However, this cultivation of pleasure and play often felt out of place in a space whose main work was remediating life's tragedies and misfortunes. On a very practical level, insurance companies frequently refused to pay for interventions that appeared to be "recreational" rather than medical, even though they took place in a medical center and were arguably the best means to remedy a medically diagnosable set of problems. So parents paid out of pocket for our social skills groups and structured activities. What they paid were sums that felt significant even to the upper middle-class clientele of the center and that were completely out of reach for less affluent families and for most adults with Asperger's living independently. The prices were nonetheless lower than what the medical center would typically be reimbursed for a similar amount of a health care provider's time prescribing medications or conducting diagnostic assessments. The finances of the center were thus an ongoing source of concern.

The Group Group also based its interventions very heavily on the positive aspects of Asperger's syndrome, seeking out and building up the common ground shared by people with the diagnosis that might make them want to spend time with each other and, ideally, make other people want to spend time with them as well. The Hayes Center, on the other hand, saw its work as mitigating the impact of negative forces, such as illness, disease, and the kinds of misbehavior thought to fall under those classifications, that one would rather eliminate entirely if one could. The Psychiatry Department building was surrounded by a series of striking, well-designed advertisements depicting childhood psychiatric disorders, including Asperger's syndrome, as malevolent entities that robbed children of their childhood. Dr. Grace found these ads not only offensive but also embarrassing; they fundamentally misrepresented the nature of her work. The depiction of Asperger's syndrome as dread disease made it seem like something you wanted to get away from as quickly as possible. But the Group Group frequently dealt in social pleasures, not social ills. The goal was to motivate desire, not avoidance; to craft activities that people would seek out and enjoy; and to create spaces that people didn't want to leave and relationships that they sought to take outside with them.

For example, the Group Group considered one of its greatest success stories to be the friendship of Angela and Rachel, the two girls in the Drama Group. After the first few weeks of the Drama Group, we noticed that the girls and their mothers were arriving at the clinic earlier and earlier and staying later and later after the workshop was finished. The mothers, thrilled at the budding friendship, allowed themselves to be dragged into the clinic early and talked together in the waiting room after the workshop while their daughters held extended playdates among the assortment of toys and board games. The Group Group watched from around the corner and exchanged quiet high fives. The rest of the psychiatry department staff, however, was perplexed and a little put off by the notion of little girls taking over the waiting room, refusing to leave the doctor's office.

"I've been doing social skills groups and training people do them and having them for pushing 20 years now," Dr. Grace told me, exasperated, in our interview several months later, "and they're always unwelcome in the medical settings because the kids get boisterous. They [the medical administrators] don't want trouble in the waiting room. . . . And I had that happen at [another psychiatric center] too. The regular psychiatry department complained about us having noisy kids. Well, of course these kids are—[It would] probably be the only social thing they had all week. They get excited about seeing each other, and then they had poor social control, and they would be silly and noisy, in the waiting room, going down the hall, whatever, and we'd get complaints about it."

Are My Friends Gonna Have to Have Two Tuberculosis Tests?

The way in which the waiting rooms and hallways functioned as contested liminal spaces between the inner sanctum of the medical center and a boisterous, messy social world is a particularly vivid example of an ongoing tension between the demands of treating Asperger's and the traditional practices of a medical center. Containing contagion, recognizing and managing traveling pathogens, and strictly maintaining the boundaries between within and without, are powerful imperatives that shape the practices of the medical setting in deep and pervasive ways. The work of the Asperger Center, with its focus on social life, challenged those imperatives by prioritizing transmission and generalization over containment and enclosure and by generally blurring the boundaries between the inside and the outside—of the clinic and of its participants.

The center's interventions often involved bringing as much as possible of the outside world into the clinic, in all its unpredictability. The greatest challenge faced by the Group Group was teaching realistic, generalizable social skills that could be flexibly adapted to a variety of settings presenting a variety of unexpected demands. We were all too familiar with kids who endlessly recited the scripts they'd learned in social skills class, even in situations when they were patently ridiculous. But realistic situations involving real people were difficult to artificially re-create: We adults, even Anna with her theater training, could only go so far with our impersonations of contemporary 9-year-olds. Our replicas and role-plays of social events—*Pretend you're going to a store! Pretend you're asking a friend to play!*—lacked the very complexity and unexpectedness that made socializing in the real world so overwhelming for the Asperger's clients. It felt a lot more effective to bring in real people who were not acting as patients or practitioners but as ordinary people you might meet out in the world: friends, teachers, ticket collectors, artistic collaborators.

However, efforts to bring in outsiders were frequently challenged by the tangled thicket of medical bureaucracy that regulated what kind of bodies and what kind of people were allowed to enter this protected space. To interact with individuals designated as patients at the clinic and to get the badge that entitled one to pass freely through the clinic (it literally as well as figuratively opened all the doors), visitors had to gain some sort of official status, usually by becoming a volunteer or staff member of the medical school. This process entailed a prolonged scrutiny of one's medical and immunity status: two tuberculosis tests (each of which required 2 visits spaced exactly 2 days apart) and a physical examination, giving a few vials of blood for analysis, filling out extensive paperwork disclosing one's entire medical and treatment history, every medication ever taken and what it was taken for. It was a whole lot of questions and a whole lot of needles, and every once in a while, something would get lost by someone somewhere and the whole process would have to start all over again. This scrutiny of the physical stuff of our bodies made perfect sense in the context of concern about the transmission of pathogens between sick patients and health care providers. When we were trying to bring in a couple of Anna's filmmaker friends to help run the filmmaking club, on the other hand, the process felt frustrating and arbitrary. "Are my friends gonna have to have two TB [tuberculosis] tests?" Anna wailed, not optimistic that they would stick it out. Such perpetual management of potential contagion served as an ongoing reminder that we were in a space of containment and control, a place whose practices are dictated by the logics of diseases in bodies. Interventions to contain transmission conflicted with interventions to encourage generalization and cross-contextual spread.

Similarly, a well-validated intervention for teaching social skills to kids with Asperger's is to involve neurotypical peers as mentors—what Tony Attwood (1997) wryly refers to as "rent-a-friend." The Group Group on several occasions discussed the possibility of inviting kids with no diagnosis into the mix of our workshops and social groups so that they could model typical social behavior. Each time, however, we were daunted by the difficulty of bringing persons who were not clearly marked as either doctor or patient across the boundaries between clinic and world. "You have to think about, like, HIPAA [Health Insurance Portability and Accountability Act], and they're not our patients, they're seeing our patients, they're not paying, why are they here, and all this silliness," Dr. Grace sighed.

These regulations she referred to—HIPAA regulations—highlighted and reinforced the conflict between the containment and the transmission of communicable things in an ongoing, subtle, but powerful way. Management of patient information in all medical treatment centers in the United States is governed by HIPAA, a set of federal regulations that regulate the privacy and portability of protected health information (PHI). PHI is any information that "relates to the individual's past, present or future physical or mental health or condition, [and/or] the provision of health care to the individual . . . for which there is reasonable basis to believe it can be used to identify the individual" (Department of Health and Human Services, n.d., p. 4). Treatment for stigmatized conditions, such as those related to HIV, substance use, and mental health, are especially closely regulated. The regulations themselves are sweeping in scope but somewhat ambiguous in their wording, and the stakes around compliance are high.

"What HIPAA means is, I'm not sure what it stands for, but what it means is this: a little thing could get you into very big trouble" is how the nervous young man from Employee Services began the required HIPAA training that was part of my volunteer orientation. "Now you work with children—you have to be extra careful what you say to children, because they have big mouths. Let's say you're talking to Bobby, he's asking lots of questions, it's better maybe not to say anything at all. Because let's say you say something to Bobby, and Bobby tells Jenny, and Jenny tells her mother, and then Jenny's not allowed to play with Bobby anymore. Even the smallest little thing you say, that's diagnosis-related, that's a HIPAA violation," he warned me sternly.

Kids' talk, the very casual conversation we sought to develop, here was depicted as highly risky for both the children and the organization—especially if it involved information about the diagnosis that served as their initial point of common ground. Health information, in this setting, functions like a disease itself: Once you come into contact with it, you must take precautions lest you spread it to others.

This policy, its ramifications, and the climate of fear and ambiguity surrounding it, all presented problems for our attempts to build a creative community of proud Asperger's artists. "They'll want to put the films up on YouTube," one of the clinicians laughed during a discussion of our nascent filmmakers' club, and then the room fell silent in sudden, shared concern. Would such public performance violate these regulations? After all, the actors, scriptwriters, and directors of this proposed piece would all share a diagnosis, and such a biosocial bond also constitutes protected health information. The experiences they shared, the circumstances and personal qualities that brought them together, might well be visible in their completed work. But we wanted our filmmakers to have the same opportunities that their neurotypical peers would have, and that included being able to share their work freely through the social media that is so much a part of contemporary social life. Similarly, Anna noted that in every drama class she had ever run, the parents circulated a contact sheet with each others' addresses and phone numbers so that they could continue to facilitate friendships between their kids outside of the program; here in a medical setting that treated social isolation, where that process would be most useful, we questioned whether such information could be freely shared. The HIPAA privacy regulations and the hospital's policies around them had been developed and implemented with a very good intention: to protect individuals from the stigma of illness. However, such practices, with their focus on the dangerousness of "health information" and all its power to harm, were not able to account for and accommodate the condition that now presented itself to the clinic staff, with its surprising valences of performance and pride.

All Films Will Be Set at the Borders

The Group Group was presented with a dilemma: the work they had been brought to the medical center to do was in many ways antithetical to the confines and structures of medical practice. The solution to this problem was often to leave the clinic—both symbolically and literally. Outside the walls of the medical center, people and information flowed more freely. While I was still in the process of getting my clearance as a volunteer, one of the social groups for adolescents, led by a therapist named Veronica, decided that their activity for that week would be to go get an ice cream from a well-known local ice cream stand. For various reasons, this was a good week for me to be introduced to the group members. I couldn't officially join the group, of course, not yet being an official volunteer, but Veronica pragmatically suggested there was nothing to stop me from deciding I wanted to buy an ice cream.

Leaving the rooms of the clinic behind meant leaving behind many structural reminders that the condition was considered an illness: the brochures on the walls discussing the tragedy of pediatric depression and Tourette's syndrome, the scales and stethoscopes lurking uselessly in the background. The members of James's Sports Talk group decided that they felt self-conscious sitting in the clinic talking about baseball and opted instead to meet at the café in a nearby Borders bookstore. After he reported this in one of our meetings, Veronica sardonically suggested that maybe the filmmaking group could meet there as well, solving some of their problems of stigma and public disclosure. "All films will be set at the Borders!" she announced grandly while the group broke into that laughter.

Our gradual move out of the medical realm of the clinic happened in our language as well as our physical location. Gradually changing the terms we used to describe ourselves and our work allowed us and those kids we now hesitated to call *patients* to pass more easily between social spaces. During one of our meetings, we figured that if Anna's filmmaker friends were operating as medical staff, interacting with patients in a clinical capacity, then they would need to go through the arduous scrutiny of the Employee Health office. If our filmmaking group was a medical intervention, then the identities of participants would need to be kept secret. But what if Anna's friends were *trainers*? Dr. Grace mused. What if Anna's group wasn't considered to be a medical intervention—what if we called it a *training*? Training, classes, and other such educational interventions occupied a subtly different status within the bureaucracy of the center, requiring different forms of documentation and staffing. Reimagining our work as nonmedical allowed us to operate around and through medical regulations, giving us justification to operate with a bit more flexibility. Language was a powerful tool for transforming our ideas of our work into something that could operate in compliance with ambiguous regulations, and the language of "training" caught on quickly as a means of distancing ourselves from medicine and its constraints.

On the last day of the Drama Group, as spring was turning into muggy summer and I was packing my bags to depart from the field, we three co-leaders mulled over a closing ceremony that would celebrate the work of all the participants. "What do they call them at trainings?" Anna asked. "Certificates of Completion. That's what we'll give them." Anna pulled out a box of certificates she had picked up at the Office Depot, labeled with little gold cups, clearly designed for the corporate setting. "*For Outstanding Work During the Month of _____*" read the template on the front of the box. And so it was that as we sang our last round of "It's Time to Say Shalom," as Angela and Rachel and Jeriah and Juan ran around the room, waving their puppets and shrieking with excitement and fear and sadness and relief at the end of things, we proudly handed them each a certificate: *For Outstanding Work During the Month of August*. Our transformation from healing practice into training activity, in all its resonances both educational and corporate, was complete.

When I returned to the city a year later for follow-up, the Asperger Center had closed. An odd fit to begin with, the program had not brought in the kind of money that the administration had hoped it would; meanwhile, the private funding had ended. Martina Grace, James, Anna, and a number of the other members of the Group Group had left the medical center entirely; Ellen (now done with her training and a fully licensed psychologist) and a few others remained at Hayes, continuing to see patients with Asperger's syndrome through the psychiatry department. As I interviewed each of them in their new settings— Martina and James in their private practices, Ellen in her office at the medical school—I observed how sharply the work of these spaces had diverged. At the medical school, treatment for Asperger's syndrome focused exclusively on the pathology of individuals; creativity, social life, and pleasure had left the building.

I Look at Them as Someone Who Has Significant Social Impairments

After the closing of the Asperger Center, Ellen remained at Hayes, hired directly into the Department of Psychiatry. She spends half of her time doing individual therapy with adolescents and the other half working on a research study on an experimental medication to treat depression. For her patients who have Asperger's, she provides mostly cognitive behavioral therapy, teaching them to adjust their thoughts and behaviors, learn new social skills, and manage their emotions to better fit their surroundings. She told me:

> I see, unfortunately, a lot of high school–aged kids [with Asperger's] that are becoming depressed and lonely and anxious because they feel—and most of the time they're right—that they don't have good social skills. And as a result, kids that used to be their friends are excluding them from groups, they're not getting invited to dances, they're getting made fun of.
>
> I have one young man who has real difficulty being aware when he has food on his face. Many times, he's had lunch in the cafeteria and he's had food on his face, and he didn't know it, and he was made fun of. So now, he's not eating lunch at school. Then he's hungry and that makes him more irritable, so he's not coping as well with stressors that normally he would cope with. So then, he'll have what his parents will call a meltdown or an outburst, and then that's more stigmatizing.

Ellen's work at the medical school, while maintaining a clear awareness of the social contexts of patients' difficulties, focuses on the individual as both the locus of the problem and the site of intervention. She teaches a kid not to have food on his face; she helps him to feel and act differently when the other kids tease him about it. If Ellen had the capacity to intervene in the social arena, she might question what is wrong with a person who turns on a friend because he has food on his face; she might question why it is OK to make fun of a kid with food on his face in the first place. But, although she may ask these questions privately, she cannot do so within the scope of her work. Her work is with the single patient, so instead the problem is his, and she works with him to solve it by better managing his depression and anxiety, teaching him not to display those feelings in stigmatizing ways. The legitimately depressing and anxiety-provoking moral truth of the world she works in is that exclusion and rejection by former friends is the natural consequence of the victim's lack of social skill.

Ellen's conception of what the disorder is—and who her patients are—is delineated by the kind of work she can do within the treatment model she occupies:

> ELLEN: When I actually work with a person in my office, I don't look at them as someone with Asperger syndrome. I look at them as someone who has significant social impairments, and we have to work on that. And I don't think: if they didn't have the social impairment, they wouldn't have the great talent in this area. I look at the person as: they have a really great talent in this area, but [the social impairment] is what we're going to focus on, because this is their weakness. I don't look at it as: it all came together as a package. . . . And there's no use for me to look at it any differently in terms of treatment. For me, treatment is based on improving the areas of deficit.

When Ellen looks at a patient, she does not see a person with Asperger's syndrome, where the syndrome is "a package" that is likely to come along with talents and strengths, because there is no use in doing so within a treatment model that is focused on improving areas of deficit. She sees a person characterized by the significant social impairments that are the focus of treatment. Although she strives to be aware of her patients' strengths and to make her patients aware of them as well, such a model allows her little room to conceptualize a consistent relationship between the strengths and impairments of the patients she treats.

As her work with patients is confined to the clinic, she cannot access the actual social spaces in which her patients' problems manifest, and this limitation frustrates her. She can teach social skills, but she doesn't know how her patients are using them outside of her office, what kind of social life these skills and practices take on outside of the dyadic conversations between doctor and patient—how well the therapy is actually working.

> ELLEN: You never know for sure if the skills are generalizing. . . .
> So say, for example [a patient] knows that every other Friday night,
> one of his colleagues goes around and asks people to go out for
> happy hour. He doesn't know if he should say yes, or how he should
> respond. And if he does say yes, [he doesn't know] how he should
> act. . . . If the patient can identify a situation like that, then we can
> role-play and we can talk about specific skills to use. We can write
> them down; he can take them with him; we can create checklists that
> he can discreetly look at when he's in a situation and monitor his
> own behavior. Those are all things that I've done to help the general-
> ization. But we actually can't be in [the situation]—I'm not at the bar
> with him, and when he comes back to me a week later and reports
> what he did, or even if he e-mails me his checklist, it's all coming
> from his perspective.

Ellen clearly cares very much for her patients. She sympathizes with their pain and the difficulty of their situation, and she is doing everything that she can to help them. She spends a great deal of time thinking about what the best way to help patients really is, reading up on the effectiveness of various interventions, and devoting half her professional hours to treatment efficacy research. She is doing the work that she has trained for many years to do, and she is very good at it. But the model within which she is working constrains her to a focus on a circumscribed slice of her patients' experience, abstracted from the worlds within which that experience takes place—a slice that contains only individual deficits and not the social injustice nor the strengths and pleasures that give that experience a richer and more livable meaning.

The Creativity That Comes with Their Wiring Differences

I met with James in the private office where he now meets with his clients; he also collaborates with colleges and universities all over the city and surrounding areas, running a program that supports high school graduates with Asperger's as they began college. He continues to see some clients individually and meets weekly with the Exploring the City group that had begun at the Asperger Center. Over the past year, the group has grown into a close-knit community of 12 young adults, exploring the vicissitudes of friendship, attraction, and adult life together.

When I asked him how he had managed to establish the kind of mutual trust he saw developing within the group, he responded that while he and his co-facilitator worked very hard to create a safe space,

> I think that just being together once a week, every week, every month, eventually people get confidence. They relax, their anxiety subsides, and we start to see who they really are. And they're wonderful people. Something that I'm always looking for when I work with people, individually or a group, is *that person*. I'm looking for creativity all the time too. I'm a big believer in creativity. I believe that most of the people that we're working with, I know that they all see the world differently, but how can that different view be used as a strength?
>
> And I find so often that they have some really special—art, music, writing, something that really can set them apart, and that when we can identify that and work with that, we can then get onto building self-esteem. Which is another huge issue, because for me they're all suffering from posttraumatic stress disorder. They have been bullied and abused and left out and made to think that they're damaged goods their whole life. . . . I think that the more that we begin to identify the creativity that comes with their wiring differences and their perceptual differences—I think that the more and sooner we do that, the better off we'll be.

James's conceptualization of his clients differs in several significant ways from Ellen's conceptualization of her patients. For one thing, discovering the ways in which his clients are "wonderful people" is not disconnected from his therapeutic work with them but is, in fact, a critical part of the work. Furthermore, the reason why it is therapeutically helpful to gradually uncover that wonderful person is because of the difficult nature of that person's social context and the cumulative effect of being mistreated and misconstrued within it over time. Here, the bullying, abuse, and being left out are not merely the direct consequences of the victim's deficits but also the moral responsibility of the abuser; the responsibility of the victim is to heal, by recognizing and reclaiming their creativity and strength.

Last, James, unlike Ellen, explicitly casts the creativity and the struggles of his Asperger's clients as part of a single package of co-occurring traits, all of which "comes with their wiring differences." James is deeply aware of the difficulties, costs, and consequences of this different wiring, telling me,

> These guys have real neurological differences. They're missing a wire that allows them to understand interpersonal relationships. They are missing through that wiring 70% of the transaction. They can't read faces most of the time. They don't read expressions. They can't read moods. They have no what we call theory of mind. Remember that one? Where I understand what you're thinking, and so I'm reacting to what I think you're thinking—[for them it's] more like a blank screen. That's a huge disadvantage.

But to James, a crucial part of both understanding people with Asperger's syndrome and addressing the problems caused by their differences is to perceive creativity, too, as part of the "wiring," an inextricable part of the package.

They're Not Patients If There's Nothing Really Wrong with Them

"I'm discarding the medical model altogether," Martina Grace told me when I called her to set up an interview. "Now I call them clients, not patients."

> I don't like calling them patients, but I got into the habit [in medical schools]. I prefer calling them clients, because they're not patients if

there's nothing really wrong with them to me. . . . If we could change our model around to where it's a health-based model, then I might not mind the medical model. But since our current medical model is illness-based—I don't think it's appropriate for people with Asperger's syndrome to think of them as ill.

In Dr. Grace's view, the medical model's exclusive focus on pathology renders it inappropriate to describe and deal with a condition such as Asperger's. Medical models also tend to support and encourage pharmacological interventions, which, in the case of Asperger's syndrome, do little to alter the core symptoms of the condition.

By emphasizing [the] medical model, we're putting Band-Aids on it by medicating them, and there's no medication for this. . . . "Oh, Ritalin didn't work." Well, of course Ritalin didn't work. They're inattentive because they're so anxious they can't get through their day, not because they have ADHD. . . . *We've tried everything.* No you haven't. You've tried medical model interventions. . . . The interventions for autism are not medical, they're educational. You are creating different cognitions, and different brain patterns, within them by the teaching.

Now, instead of relying on a neurochemical model centered around medications, she offers coaching, transition planning around going away to college, social skills seminars, training for parents on how to set up effective, activity-filled playdates for their kids—education about how to live effectively out in the world. Such educational practices, as she noted, do "create different brain patterns" in individuals, but they do so by engaging with not only the brains of individuals but also the social context in which those individuals are embedded.

Her work, like James's, thus demands engagement with *the package*: with both the individual *and* the social challenges *and* gifts that come with Asperger's syndrome. For example, understanding and effectively addressing her clients' problems with employment involves understanding the challenges posed by their strengths as well as by their weaknesses, in the context of the particular demands of the entry-level work that is frequently their lot at the lowest rungs of the social ladder:

Work in McDonald's is *malemployment*. It's not just *under*[employment], of course it's *under*[employment], but it's also *mal*[employment] because it's demanding socially and not demanding intellectually. Lots of entry-level jobs are like that.[1]

Her understanding of the current prevalence of Asperger's as well as its role in society draws on an awareness of the physiological and the sociological history of certain correlated traits. She wonders, for example, whether the high rates of Asperger's she has observed among her Jewish clients is due not only to the high levels of professional help seeking she has observed in that population overall but also due to the genetic impact of the social valuation of certain Asperger's cognitive traits, going all the way back to the Middle Ages:

> The best yeshiva boy, the smartest yeshiva boy—and many of those characteristics that would make you good at studying little teensy pieces of the Torah and stuff, stuff that would make you good at that, are also characteristics that are often found in Asperger's syndrome—they would arrange [for him to] marry the daughter of the well-to-do guy of the well-to-do family in town. And guess what? Those children [of well-to-do parents] *lived* more, in the 1300 and 1400s. So they did selective breeding!

Thus, understanding the current prevalence of Asperger's requires understanding that certain traits have a genetically transmissible coexistence that is completely independent of the shifting sociohistorical contexts in which these traits take on their socially valued or devalued meanings. This physiologically rooted "package" of interlinked characteristics exists independently from societal judgments about what constitutes a deficit at any given time and from what manifests as impairment in any given context. Yet the fact that individual elements of this consistent package of traits can be socially valued as well as devalued is also a critical explanatory component of their continued presence and prevalence.

When Dr. Grace talks about Asperger's, she describes a complex social, historical, and genetic phenomenon whose prevalence, meaning, and impact can only be understood by looking at the interweaving of characteristics, both valued and devalued, across time and social contexts. But this complex conceptualization is not one she feels she can act on within the illness-based medical model she finds in clinical settings. Her work has left the clinic with her, and left an impoverished model of patient, syndrome, and treatment behind, in which both patients and their disorders are represented by a version of themselves made up of only the impairments of their bodies.

Are You Going to Have Another Party?

While I have focused here on the experiences of one particular group in one particular place, practitioners I interviewed in a number of settings observed that the needs of clients with Asperger's stretch the constraints of traditional clinical practice. For example, while I was working in Brookfield, I had the opportunity to interview Dr. Cora Starkey, widely considered to be the region's best psychologist when it came to working with people with Asperger's. As we concluded the interview, she shared a set of concerns strikingly similar to those I heard at the Asperger Center, despite the significant differences between her rural private practice and the complex infrastructure of the urban Hayes Center:

> I trained as a clinical psychologist, y'know? And it's all, privacy this, HIPAA that, and you can't let this person know this, or that. But last week I had a potluck for my clients on the spectrum and their families. And it was at my house.
>
> I know the people who trained me wouldn't approve. You're not supposed to let patients know this or that about you. But with this population, with people on the spectrum, it's so important to build community. These parents need to be able to go to parties. And the children! One of my teenage patients said to me: are you going to have another party?
>
> I think that's where I'm going, more and more. I wouldn't do this for my more clinical patients—like, my patients with anxiety. But people on the spectrum need this kind of community building work. It's not that I have no therapeutic boundaries. I'm not inviting them to *my* birthday party. But that flexibility—I think some clinical people would think it was pretty sketchy. I don't know.

Despite her awareness of the healing power of her potluck parties, the way in which they meet the needs of both her clients and the social and family systems from which they are inextricable, Dr. Starkey still clearly feels some ambivalence about the way in which community-building challenges traditional clinical boundaries.

Dr. Starkey's struggle and the story of the Asperger Center are both part of a broader picture. The practice of medicine has expanded into new domains of social life via one paradigm—what I have been calling the "package" model of neurodevelopmental disorder—then contracted through the application of another—what I have been calling the "pathogen" model. At the Hayes Center, bureaucratic imperatives and financial incentives were organized around individual bounded bodies and other such impermeable spaces. Within such tightly regulated borders, there was no way to conceptualize Asperger's syndrome as a thing that happens not only within but also between people or to address it through the forging and management of relationships and robust, if temporary, social cultures. The infrastructure of the Hayes Center could not contain the elements of Asperger's syndrome that make it a new kind of condition: its valued aspects, its aesthetic resonances, and its irreducible engagement with the givens of the social world. In the end, these aspects of Asperger's that did not fit within the medical paradigm slipped out of those bounds rather than expanding them. Meaning, aesthetics, pleasure, and sociality return to the province of recreation, education, and the real-world life of bars and bowling alleys, and the clinic is left to manage only the individual, negative, and containable elements of autism spectrum disorders that can be easily conceptualized as "disease." The clinic is left with a medical model of Asperger's syndrome that is strikingly incomplete, that attends only to the illness-like pathologies of individual bodies, and that cannot see all the rest of it.

The story of the Hayes Center presents a case study of a wider phenomenon: the process of expansion and constriction through which arenas of human experience that transcend the borders of the individual body—aesthetics, pleasure, sociality, and our co-constitutive participation in meaningful worlds—are evoked through inclusive models of neurodevelopmental difference and then reduced back down to discrete disease entities. Such practices instantiate a conceptualization of social engagements as potentially contaminating entities that must be extruded from sharply bounded systems: from the body to the building, all the way up to society itself (see also Avery, 2020). They center the individual as the locus of agency for broader social patterns and practices. And they further entrench a model of the individual as a sharply bounded system, to whose well-being broader social forces are only tangentially relevant. As we will see in the next chapter, this conception of the person as limited to what lies within the boundaries of the body produces an intractable ethical dilemma around fiercely contested questions of prevention and cure.

7

The Dilemma of Cure

That Certain Special Thing About Trevor

"My mind is really strange," 17-year-old Trevor Trent explains to me in a tone of rueful pride. I have just asked him about his diagnosis and how he reacted to receiving it. "So I took it apart to what it sounds like: Do I get a side of fries with that? Does it come with a large or medium Coke?"

"Fries?" I ask him, confused.

"With the *ass burgers!*"

Trevor is a wit, an active participant in the insult battles that fill his classroom at ASPEN. For Trevor, this wacky, associative humor is what Asperger's syndrome is all about. "Most people tend to do the same thing with their lives, over, and over, and over. And that's lacking creativity. You gotta mix it up, you know. And us in the ASPEN program, we're always mixing it up. We all have a really twisted, yet great, sense of humor. Maybe Asperger's has something that creates something in our mind, maybe, that wants us to achieve a higher understanding of creativity, and make up for something we're either missing or have too much of." His ambition to be a writer, his obsession with odd juxtapositions of pop-cultural detritus, the assemblages and deconstructions that channel his creative energy are all inextricably tied to his condition.

For Trevor's stepfather, on the other hand, the Asperger's diagnosis means something very different: It provides a biological explanation that helps him cope with how infuriating Trevor can be to deal with. Seemingly oblivious to the niceties of social propriety, Trevor has a tendency to say exactly what's on his mind, regardless of the context. When he is engrossed in one of the comic books he obsessively reads and collects, getting his attention for anything else—dinnertime, bedtime, the needs of others—is nearly impossible. Sloppy with his own work, he flies into perfectionistic rages at other people's departures from form, once threatening his brother with a knife for mispronouncing the name of a character from *Star Wars*.

At first, Mr. Trent took this as a reflection on Trevor's character. But then the diagnosis, he told me, "gave me an answer to *why doesn't he get it*, especially with things regarding interactions with other people and certain accepted norms, things you do, things you don't do in interacting with people. And so realizing that there was something more behind it, other than just a conscious decision on his part, made it a little bit easier."

Thinking of Asperger's as a disease has allowed Mr. Trent to draw a sharp separation between Trevor's exasperating, insulting behaviors and Trevor himself, a separation that makes it easier for him to treat his stepson with respect, patience, and love. "I was able to [say]—*OK, it's not you, it's the behavior. It's not you, it's the disease*—and look at it and say OK, maybe this is happening because of the Asperger's and maybe I need to look at things a little bit differently." This perspective makes it possible for him to imagine a Trevor without Asperger's, a Trevor who has kept all his talents and interests but lost the impediments to their expression. "He's very skilled. He's very talented. He writes amazing stories, he can compose music. I mean, he's very, very talented. And he enjoys it. I get the feeling that if he didn't have all these other things going on in his head, if he didn't have all these other issues that he was trying to deal with, I think he would have gained skills that would have helped him apply himself and put things together."

If there were a cure for Asperger's, I asked him, would he want Trevor to take it? "In a heartbeat. To be able to see him take these things and kind of put them all together and run with it, that would be great. And I have to imagine that he'd probably opt to change it himself if he could. Trevor hasn't had an easy time."

Trevor, however, answers that question very differently than his stepfather imagines. When I ask him if he would go back in time, if he could, and make it so that he didn't have Asperger's, he tells me about a classroom assignment he'd aced, years ago, on *Lord of the Flies*. "I was asked: if you could take away any human emotion, what would you? And I said, 'none.' No one else said this, but I said, 'none,' because that emotion is what makes us human. Having all these emotions is what makes us human. So taking away from us, we'd not be humans anymore. That's what defines us." To Trevor, Asperger's is an element of what makes him who he is. "Maybe it's the way I think, and the way I am, my process of thinking. It defines me. It's one of the characteristics that define me and make me who I am." Within Trevor's conception of personhood, taking away a characteristic that defines him would negate the whole of his humanity.

Trevor's mother hovers between these two understandings of Asperger's: as something that can be separated from Trevor or as something that cannot, something that impedes his personhood or something that instantiates it. "I wish there was a cure for it," she sighed. But when I asked her what she thought a cure would do for him, she replied, "It would probably make him feel more accepted. But in a sense, it would take away that certain special thing about Trevor. I don't know."

Mrs. Trent has good reason to worry about Trevor's future. As he prepares to turn 18 and graduate from the public high school system into abrupt adulthood, his family is facing a question that will determine much of the course of the rest of his life: Can he live independently? "He's going to be 18 in October. And the long-standing joke was that when you're 18, you're out of here," Mrs. Trent told me. "And I don't see that happening." She worries about how he will fare on his own when he still needs so many reminders to get up in the morning, to go to bed at night, to complete and turn in his work. She worries about how he will get and keep a job in a tight employment market that prioritizes soft skills—communication skills, time management, teamwork—when he doesn't pay attention to things that aren't interesting to him and doesn't seem to get that he shouldn't insult his boss like he insults his peers. "He doesn't even have a job. He's 17. When I was 15, I had a job, I had a car, I had—and it's so different. He had a job for a short time and it didn't last . . ." Trevor's school is beginning to ask difficult questions about whether he will be able to live independently at all, proposing that the family apply for a range of disability support services, raising the possibility of a group home. Mrs. Trent has begun watching the developmentally disabled man who bags groceries at her local supermarket under a supported employment program, wondering if this is the future of her clever, creative son.

Even as she is aware of the cost of Trevor's condition, she has a hard time imagining, as her husband does, a sharp separation between the condition and Trevor. She describes Asperger's as "a disease that affects my son's thinking, his ability to function socially" but, at the same time, sees it as a constitutive part of who he is, part of Trevor's essential Trevor-ness. She deeply values that particularity, even as she recognizes that Trevor's idiosyncratic way of being will make it difficult for him to function as an adult in his world. He is coming of age in a society in which such specificity of self is valued and cultivated and in which independence is prized as a measure of success. Yet it is also one in which that independence can be acquired only by playing very well with others: through flexible cooperation and fluent compliance with social norms. This irony puts his mother in a moral quandary. Would a cure be worth it to her, I ask, if it worked as she imagined: made him fit in better but took away "that certain special thing"?

"Yes and no" she replies, tearing up. "I don't know how to answer that question."

Within one family, Asperger's syndrome was three different things. To Trevor, it was an intrinsic part of his human nature; to his stepfather, it was a disease, separate from and antithetical to Trevor's development as a person; to his mother, it was a part of Trevor's unique individuality but one that paradoxically threatened his ability to function as an individual unsupported by family or society. Trevor did not want to be cured of his condition, Mr. Trent embraced the idea of a cure and assumed Trevor would too, and his mother was painfully uncertain. These different ways of understanding Asperger's syndrome have powerfully shaped Trevor's life and the lives of his family. When I returned to Brookfield a year after these first interviews, his mother and stepfather had separated, in large part due to deep disagreements over what to expect from him.

When I began the research that led to this book, I was perplexed, inspired, and intrigued by the questions being posed within the autism community about cure, prevention, and their implications. What would a cure for autism do? What are the stakes of developing a preventative intervention for a condition whose very definition is indeterminate, in constant flux? How had these questions of cure and prevention so thoroughly divided the public face of the autism community, driving wedges between advocacy groups led by parents, doctors, and researchers and those led by autistic self-advocates? How are these divisions affecting those coming of age under such contested descriptions? I had a feeling that there was more to the moral conflict of cure than was clearly visible through the polarizations of public rhetoric and that some insight could be found within the daily life negotiations of those most immediately affected: people on the autism spectrum, their families, and those whose work is dedicated to their well-being.

I was intrigued by these questions not only because I was interested in the different ways of conceptualizing autism—as a disease, as an identity, as something else entirely—but also because this issue speaks to broader questions about what makes us who we are. Alice, Trevor's teacher in the senior high school classroom at ASPEN, knows this well. When I asked for her feelings and opinions about a cure for autism, she told me about how autism fascinated her and how her work with people on the spectrum had changed her in ways she deeply appreciated. Then she acknowledged the intensity of her students' struggles, their discomforts, their thwarted longings, and their unmet needs. In the end, the question she grappled with transcended such cost–benefit calculations. "It is hard," she mused. "Because you're talking sort of fundamentally about *what is a person*, you know?"

Such philosophical questions are navigated every day in the hearth and hearts of the families of Brookfield, as they sort out the complexities of what it means to care. These negotiations play out in classrooms, in clinics, and in research laboratories, but they start in the intimate space of the family, so this chapter, which takes up these questions most directly, takes place there as well.

I Think You Should Be Asking About Parental Relationships

Disagreements about autism in the public sphere—about what it is, about what should be done about it—often seem to play out across generational divides, pitting a predominantly youthful group of autistic self-advocates against a parental-medical establishment exemplified by organizations such as Autism Speaks. Part of this schism, as previous chapters have explored, has to do with shifting paradigms in psychiatric medicine. As new generations come of age under the description of autism, they find themselves living under different descriptions than those their parents had known, with different understandings of the relationships between person and disorder. As older conceptualizations of psychiatric disorder as pathogen-like disease overlap uneasily with newer conceptualizations of psychiatric disorders as disturbances in the circuitry that constitutes the self, those who grew up with these different ideas also struggle to reconcile their approaches to autism. This can lead to differences of opinion between parents who want a cure for autism and children who do not.

During my interview with Burke's mother, Callie, Burke (who had initially shown little interest in being interviewed) overheard our conversation, came over, and joined in. In response to my interview questions, they started hashing out their different perspectives on what autism is and what a cure would do.

> ELIZABETH (TO CALLIE): How do you think the world would be different if there were a cure for autism?
>
> CALLIE: A lot smarter people in the world, that's for sure.
>
> BURKE: No. Actually most of the autistic people, actually, are smarter than most people.
>
> CALLIE: That's what I said. There would be more smart people in the world.
>
> BURKE: You're saying an oxymoron. You just said autistic people are smart.
>
> CALLIE: They are.
>
> BURKE: If you got rid of autism, where are the smart people that were autistic?
>
> CALLIE: They'll still be smart.
>
> BURKE: You can't cure it like that, technically.
>
> CALLIE: Why?
>
> BURKE: It's hereditary. You can't kill the gene inside of somebody, basically, wipe that out because it'll screw up their DNA and pretty much destroy them. The baby is born autistic, so you have to get rid of the gene before the baby is born. So if you do that, the baby don't have autism. That means the baby ain't smart. [To me] I confused the hell out of her.
>
> CALLIE: You did.

But while there is confusion in their conversation with each other, both of their perspectives make complete sense within the paradigms through which each of them learned to think about autism. Callie, here, is talking about autism like a pathogen. Even as she concurs with Burke that autistic people may be, on the whole, smarter than most, she still conceives of autism itself as being separable from both those people and those abilities. Thus, a cure for autism would allow them to function better while leaving their smartness intact. Burke, on the other hand, has learned to think of autism according to a different model, as an emergent and multivalent aspect of an interlinked genetic system. The fundamental nature of the entire system is changed if any one element of it is changed, and to change a person in this way would be to "pretty much destroy them." The only way to prevent autism, then, is to preemptively "get rid of the gene before the baby is born," thus eliminating everything that autism is, including the smartness.

When debates over a cure for autism often split between parent advocacy groups and autistic self-advocates, however, it is the result of more than just this generational gap in medical metaphors. The intergenerational dynamics of autistic self-advocacy, the right of autistic people to determine their own life pathways according to their own wants, needs, and desires, is also complicated by family histories. Most parents raising a child on the autism spectrum have spent a great deal of time and effort, throughout that child's life, trying to get them to stop doing things they want to do and to do things they don't want to do instead. Parent–child relationships are thus often characterized, even more so than in families unaffected by autism, by an ongoing battle of wills over autonomy, safety, and the determinants of well-being.

Lyndon is a college senior I met through the ASPNET support groups. I asked him, as I usually do at the end of each interview, whether there was anything I should be asking about that I hadn't asked. Lyndon responded right away:

> I think you should be asking about parental relationships. For me at least it's been a pretty darn important aspect of how I became who I am. According to my therapist, she goes to these meetings for, like, parents with kids with disabilities and like, you know, it's *parents and kids with Asperger's get very, very, very intertwined.* You know it's—I don't want to quite call it an enmeshed family relationship, but I think on some level it is.

I asked him why he thought this was. He replied:

> Well, if you have a parent who cares, I think it's just concern. It's like: *My God, is this kid gonna be OK?* You know, and you have to make sure every second. You know, like: *Is he gonna be OK? Is he OK? Is he OK? Is he crazy?* I don't know firsthand. I've never asked my parents, but I think that probably has a little something to do with it. I think there's an element there, like it's simultaneously kind of concern and fear and shame and pride. You know? Maybe I'm being presumptuous but I feel like there's so many complicated emotions attached to what's happening to your son.

Lyndon was doing well in a highly selective college, after a childhood of special education services, intensive psychotherapy, and fairly constant intervention in his social life by his parents. His diagnosis had transformed the life of his mother, who left her teaching job to become a full-time professional advocate for students with disabilities. "I mean everything with my mother has just been, like, an ordeal when it comes to this," he told me. "It's either an advocacy session or it's, like, an instructorial session, and I think right now what we're trying to work on is making it a bit more like a—we're trying to have a bit more of a familial relationship as opposed to, you know, this complicated familial intertwined with business."

But he recognizes that, to a certain extent, this degree of parental involvement has kept him moving forward in the world. "I mean I get down on my parents for being so hard on me, but on some level I think if they weren't so hard on me I wouldn't do anything with my life. 'Cause I wouldn't know how to. I'd just sit at home playing Scrabble on Facebook all the time."

This is a realistic concern. For youth on the spectrum, their tendency toward intense focus makes them particularly susceptible to technologies designed to capture attention and exploit it for commercial profit—video games, collectible cards, YouTube channels. Social participation in an uncongenial world of jobs and teachers and peers often feels hopeless and unmotivating, especially compared to the pursuit of deep interests that produce a sense of self-efficacy and mastery. Sensory sensitivities make many self-care activities such as dressing and showering dramatically less appealing than other forms of sensory stimulation or

avoidance. Yet giving in to the desire to stay in pajamas all day playing Minecraft or researching World War II aircraft means missing out
on the kind of life opportunities—jobs, education, socialization outside
the home—generally thought to contribute to social inclusion and long-
term success.

Earlier in this book, we met Andrew Yollen, a recent high school
graduate whose focus on his interests and desires was strong enough
to tax even the energy, ingenuity, and patience of the Journeyfolk camp
counselors. Andrew's pattern of allocating energy to the activities that
capture his attention, at the expense of more tedious expectations such
as chores and hygiene, created constant battles with his father and step-
mother, who were raising him. Mr. Yollen, who works nights, told me,

> I'll get home from work, and at 8:30, 9:00 in the morning, I'm like: *You
> know what? It's time to get up.* So I make him get up. We tell him to do his
> laundry. We still have to tell him to take his medicine. Deodorant, brush
> his teeth. The only thing he'll do regularly, he'll take his own shower. But I
> swear, sometimes I think he just stands in there—stands in the water, and
> gets out again. Personal hygiene is definitely a problem.

When he cleans out the cat's litterbox, it still smells. When his father gives
him money for food at the start of the week, he spends it all on candy and
soda within the first few days. The conflicts are constant and wearing.

But if he didn't push, Mr. Yollen is afraid Andrew would turn out like
his friend Cory who lives down the road. Cory, like Andrew, is on the
autism spectrum, but unlike Andrew, he doesn't have a job, and as far
as Mr. Yollen can see, he spends most of every day in his room, playing
video games. "If we did not push him, that is exactly what he would do.
He would sit down in his room with his Game Boy or a TV, and he would
not leave the house. I'm telling you, he wouldn't leave." So he keeps on
pushing against the tidal force of Andrew's attention and its tendency to
gravitate inexorably toward the seductions of the video games and the
candy and the fantasy—getting Andrew to go outside, to get a job, to keep
moving. And the results have been encouraging. When I last saw Andrew, he was in a job training program that balanced high expectations
with abundant support, and he was thriving there. "You got to push him
constantly. It pisses him off, but I do it every single day anyway."

Mr. Yollen engages in these constant battles of will, as exhausting as they are, out of a concern for how Andrew will function as an independent adult and an awareness that his son's deviations from societal expectations put him at risk of social abandonment:

> He does—definitely has normal traits. He knows how to dress himself; he knows how to put his clothes on. He knows how to comb his hair, but doesn't do it. But he knows how to do it. He knows how to brush his teeth. You got to get on him. I don't think he could live by himself, and take care of himself. Not to a standard where he'd be accepted, you know what I mean?

And that fear, that Andrew will not be accepted, weighs heavily on him. When I asked Mr. Yollen if he would go back in time and make it so Andrew had never developed Asperger's syndrome, he responded,

> Yeah, I would do it tomorrow. I would do it right now, if they said, I can go back to when he was 4 years old, and avoid this, I absolutely would. Just so he could have a normal life. And face it, I'm not gonna be around forever. If something happened to me on my way to work, on the way home, or something tomorrow, what would happen with him? I don't know what would happen. He would probably become—he would get put into the county system, and be one of those guys you see riding around town. That guy who rides around on a bicycle all the time; everybody says he's a fruitcake, or a weirdo, *look at that guy*. He's getting by, he's collecting money, he's living, but that's—I think that's how he would end up. He would be cast away, cast off.

When I asked Andrew the same question, if he would go back in time and make it so he didn't have Asperger's, he gave a very different response. "I mean, it's nothing to be ashamed of," he replied. "So why would I want to? Why would I wanna go back and change myself? Be proud of who you are. I have Asperger's and I'm proud. I'm not ashamed of it. I'm not gonna hide myself away because of it." Similarly, when I asked him if he would take a cure for Asperger's if someone came up with one, he replied, "Probably not. Because then that proves that you're ashamed of what you are. Like, if you're ashamed of having autism, then you'd take a cure. But if you're like me, just hold your head up high and be like, you know what? I have it. Whatever." For Andrew, Asperger's was an issue of individual pride in himself and his particularities. For his father, Asperger's was an impediment to social personhood. And his constant work protecting Andrew from banishment to the fringes of society keeps him seeing it that way.

As Lyndon astutely observed (and as Silverman, 2012, has empathetically explored), debates over the meaning of autism, particularly around questions of prevention and cure, are deeply bound up in the dynamics of such familial relationships. Families affected by autism engage in constant negotiations to balance respect for individual autonomy with the ever-lurking potential for social abandonment, the risk of being "cast away, cast off."

In doing so, they are negotiating not only their own particular circumstances but also, I hope to show here, a fundamental problem with the conceptualization of self within which they are operating: a crisis at the heart of hyper-individualized personhood. Bellah, Madsen, Sullivan, Swidler, and Tipton (1985), in *Habits of the Heart: Individualism and Commitment in American Life*, refer to this problem as "the tendency of individualism to destroy its own conditions" (p. 150). By "individualism," they mean what they call "radical" or "ontological individualism, the idea that the individual is the only firm reality" (Bellah et al., 1985, p. 276). This understanding of the self is grounded in what Hazel Markus and Shinobu Kitayama (1991), in a classic article positing a range of possibilities for "independent" and "interdependent" selves, describe as "the so-called Western view of the individual as an independent, self-contained, autonomous entity who (a) comprises a unique configuration of internal attributes (e.g., traits, abilities, motives, and values) and (b) behaves primarily as a consequence of these internal attributes" (p. 224). But a transformation and intensification of such individualist self-organization result when social structures are dismantled or concealed through an ideology that insists they be treated as irrelevant to our sense of who we are. As discussed in earlier chapters, social theorists such as Ulrich Beck and Elisabeth Beck-Gernsheim (2002) argue that understanding oneself as disembedded from any networks of social ties has increasingly become not merely a seductive option but an imperative within the large-scale bureaucracies that structure late modern life.

Those who do not manage to function as fully independent and autonomous builders of their own biographies risk falling through the cracks and becoming one of the growing numbers of people who are dismissed from society entirely, unable to win themselves a place. Their particularities become untenable, invisible. When our vision of ourselves as individuals obscures our awareness of ourselves in our social context, we become less able to live by an ethic that values individuals. The dilemma of a cure for autism brings this issue into sharp relief.

This chapter explores the implications of such a model of the self for the ethics of response to autism and other forms of neurodevelopmental variation. The intractable quality of debates over prevention and cure arises from the fracture lines in an increasingly unsustainable concept of the self estranged from its extrasomatic context. When we view the self as a contained system, defined only by its own internal traits and the internalized traces of its history, abstracted from wider networks of social ties, then the idea of biological intervention on these aspects of the self can easily be interpreted and experienced as a profound and annihilating violation. But when social personhood is highly contingent on individual performance of particular characteristics and capacities, without respect for the broader ties between the person and their world, autistic lives can easily come to feel impossible, unthinkable, and nearly unimaginable. We thus become entrenched in moral conflict around the possibility of prevention and cure.

What follows is a discussion of these issues, as they emerged in response to a particular set of questions. I asked each research participant these questions, in some form, in each interview. These were the questions that started me off on this project, the questions that seemed to be at the heart of the conflicts dividing the autism community. They were harder questions than I knew:

How would the world be different without Asperger's/autism?
How would you/your child/your students/your patients be different?
What do you think would change if you could make it go away somehow?

And often the most difficult question of all:

If you could, would you?

We Need Special People to Spruce Shit Up

When I asked these questions of people affected by Asperger's syndrome and related autism spectrum conditions—about what the world would be like without these conditions, whether we should be looking for a cure, and how they or their families or their lives would be different without it—I got a wide variety of answers. But these answers tended to fall into a few recognizable categories.

Among those who said they would not want to see Asperger's syndrome prevented or cured, many brought up the ways in which autistic difference could be productive. They mentioned the talents and gifts that can come with it, often referencing famous inventors whose cognitive differences led to the development of new technologies or great thinkers whose outside-the-box thinking had advanced the sciences in dramatic ways. For example, when I asked Don Smith, whose son, Matthew, was then a 14-year-old in the younger classroom at ASPEN, how the world might be different without Asperger's syndrome, he replied,

> I think we would've missed a lot of stuff. They're very sharp people. They talk about Bill Gates [as having Asperger's]. Edison. Just different people like that who sit and think. They come up with different ways to deal with things. I think we would've missed a lot.

Others discussed the ways in which difference is beneficial not only because of the ways it advances normative societal goals but also because of the ways it can challenge them. As Burke put it,

> In my eyes, it's kinda stupid to try to find a cure for autism because what's really the point, in my opinion. Because if you do that, everybody's gonna act totally normal, and it's gonna be a bunch of nitpicky people now. Because, it's basically, you're gonna be—everybody's perfect. It's gonna turn into this perfect society, blah, blah, blah, blah, blah, blah, bull crap. Like that.
>
> ELIZABETH: Why do you think that would be bad, if we had a perfect society?
>
> BURKE: That's boring. We need special people to spruce shit up.

Some suggested that the process of accommodation to difference brings its own rewards. For example, Greg's mother told me:

> There's some reason that these kids are here and they're given to people. There's some reason. I don't know what it is, but someday I think we'll figure it out. I really do. No, we need people like him. We need kids like him. We do. It makes you remember that everyone's a little different, and they don't all need to be little soldiers in a classroom.

Embracing Asperger's also sometimes served as a form of social critique, a rejection of what passes for normal. Matthew's mother, Margaret Smith, works at the local supermarket, where she has plenty of opportunities to interact with typically developing teens—and she is not impressed. When I asked her how Matthew might be different if he didn't have Asperger's, she replied,

> We've discussed this different times: *Would we want him any other way?* I don't think I would want him any other way, except for the fact that it would be easier for him probably. If he was one of the regular kids out there, listening to that crappy music and wearing those droopy pants and being a smart-aleck with a dirty mouth, I don't think I'd want that way. Because he thinks all of that stuff is wrong. He thinks the music's bad. He can't understand why people wanna walk around with their underwear hanging out. He doesn't go for swearing. And working with teenagers all the time, I wouldn't want him to be like them. I find them to be really irritating. Well, he's irritating too. No, I—maybe he's better this way.

You Love the Kid for Who He Is

But overall, the most frequent response I got to these kinds of questions was some variant of the idea that without Asperger's, affected people would not be who they were—they would be someone else instead. Being a loving, appreciative parent often seemed to entail rejecting such a possibility as deeply undesirable—especially, it seemed, for mothers. For example, despite all the struggles Allen's family had been through, when I asked his mother Corinne if she would go back in time and make it so he didn't have Asperger's, she promptly responded "No, I wouldn't.

Then he wouldn't be who he is. He's perfect the way he is. No, I wouldn't change it."

This understanding of "who he is" articulates a very specific model of what it is to be a person. If Allen didn't have Asperger's, he would still be the son of Corinne, the grandson of her mother and the nephew of her sister. He would still be a citizen of the United States, a student in the Brookfield school district, an 11-year-old kid on his street in their small town. Chances are he would still be tall for his age, with the same lanky limbs and shining brown curls. But none of those things, according to Corinne and the model of personhood within which she operates, make up who he is. Instead, it is the kinds of internal characteristics described by the Asperger's diagnosis—his temperament, his preferences, his predispositions and tendencies—that define him. And there is a perfection, in his mother's eyes, to that particularity.

Similarly, when I asked Darren's mother Lindy how she thought Darren would be different if she could go back in time and make it so that he didn't have Asperger's anymore, she replied, "I can't imagine him being different. He'd be a different kid. I can't imagine Darren being any other way. This is how he is. If he wasn't Asperger's, he would be somebody completely different. Like if I had a third child, that would be my third child. He wouldn't have any of the same things he's got now. 'Cause he really is defined by his Asperger's, with what he does. The obsession with computers, the ability to sit down and do something like that for a lengthy period until it's done right. Yeah, he wouldn't be him."

"Would you do it, if you could?" I asked her.

"No, no," she replied. "You love the kid for who he is."

Lindy's second-person response to my question—"you love the kid for who he is"—highlights the way in which she is describing not only a personal experience but also a normative injunction. This is just *what you do.* Loving the kid for who he is—and not wanting him to be any different—feels like a moral and ethical imperative.

Quote Me as Saying I Want a Pill

The parents I interviewed were well aware of this moral imperative and its relevance to my research project. When they mentioned an interest in cure or prevention, it was often with hesitance, a rueful smile, or a slightly rebellious tone, all referencing the way in which their comments went against a perceived grain.

"Am I one of the only moms you met who said they'd undo it if they could?" Kevin's mother, Laurie, asked me, tentatively, near the end of our first interview. Kevin had been diagnosed with Asperger's 2 years before. He was in a state of constant conflict with his teachers at school, and the situation was wearing everybody down. Laurie was at the time struggling to decide whether to homeschool him just as she had been offered a demanding professional opportunity she had always wanted. It was a difficult time. I told her that she was not the only one.

"OK, good," she replied. "Because, you know, I read about these moms who are like so 100% accepting, and I'm still not, and it's 2 solid years now that I've known. There are moms who talk about it [the] same as if they're just talking about their kids' hair color, and I don't know how they do it, and I wish I could."

The parents I interviewed were well aware of the discourse of autism acceptance, as a form of both respect for people on the autism spectrum and appreciation for their potential contributions. Sometimes they talked about it as a discourse that felt oppressive, and the expression of alternate stances took on a defiant quality. Sarah, for example, is the mother of a man who has been professionally successful in a field where his eccentricities are tolerated; however, he has been deeply socially isolated for his entire life. Although he has never been formally diagnosed with Asperger's, and he himself rejects the diagnosis, she became captivated enough with the diagnosis and its explanatory power in her family life that she started a second career working with youth on the autism spectrum in Park City. Her interest in autism, however, has not led her to cherish it:

> I have read the political or the philosophical notion that this is wonderful. I mean, this is how you get the Bill Gates and the Einsteins of the world. Speaking as a parent, I don't need an Einstein. I need a healthy kid who is going through the stages of life feeling productive, not feeling a hell of a lot of psychic pain, not wondering why he can't get a date, and all the things that I know are causing him pain in many areas for which he has no answers.
>
> So, yeah, you know, I forego having Einstein as a son. I'm not one of these people who thinks, oh, this is wonderful, look at the contribution

they're making to society. Yeah, at what cost? You know, so: *no*. I hope they find it, and I hope they find the pill, you know, and get rid of it. Quote me as saying I want a pill. It's not fun. It's a lot of pain.

During the decade I worked on this research, I felt something shift in the social normativity of what Nick Walker (2013) calls "the neurodiversity paradigm": the idea that neurodiversity, including autism, is "a natural, healthy and valuable form of human diversity" (para. 12) and that pathologizing autism is as inaccurate and harmful as other kinds of prejudice such as racism or sexism. When I began my research, this paradigm felt like a radical and novel way of thinking; by the time I finished my interviews, it had started to feel obligatory, at least in the circles I traveled, to offer some recognition of the value of autistic cognitive diversity and to the ethical complexities of prevention and cure. Yet this increased expression of appreciation for a specific autistic style, in and of itself, was not translating on a broad scale into the kind of support that would make autistic lives fuller and easier to live. Appreciation for individual particularities was not enough.

At times, I was aware of the way in which my own research, the kinds of conversations my questions catalyzed, were contributing to this discursive shift. When I returned to visit Matthew's family several years later, his father told me that my questions had introduced him and members of his community to a new way of thinking. He described a conversation he had with a woman in their neighborhood who was raising three children on the autism spectrum:

> The question you asked last time—I've actually said this to a couple of people. I said: "I was asked a question by a girl who was doing her doctorate, who came and talked to us. And her question was, *If you could change him, so he was like normal, would you do it?* And I said, no. No. He wouldn't be the *same.*" And [the woman raising children on the spectrum] goes: "Yeah you're right! He wouldn't be the same person." So that was an awesome question. 'Cause you're like, *whoa*. Y'know?

It's a powerful idea. But on its own, it can leave us in a terrible ethical conflict, one I only really began to understand once I got to know Thomas Stevenson and his mother.

I Think He's Going to Need Help

When I first met Thomas, he was a freshman, the new kid at Valley View, and at the bottom of the classroom pecking order. The other kids resented his heavy-handed moralizing and teased him about his anxious, repetitive questions. He tended to spill things a lot. Born extremely premature, he had had a childhood full of surgeries, medications, and medical problems with often embarrassing symptoms. He had been through many different schools, including one where the violence he saw and experienced led him into near-suicidal despair. Once he got to Valley View, however, Kirk had recognized his intense interest in history and had set him to writing biographies of famous people who might have been on the autism spectrum, which he did with aplomb. And Thomas and I became pretty good friends. Despite our differences, we had a lot in common. We were both on the fringes of things, socially; we both wanted to become university professors. I also spill things a lot. When he saw me on the sidelines looking lonely, he would come over and talk to me about the travails of academia.

As supportive as I felt of Thomas's dreams, the ivory tower felt very far off. "I think he's going to need help," his mother, Mrs. Stevenson, told me in our interview.

> I think he might be able to have a job, and I certainly hope, but he's going to need help. He's not going to be a person that's just going to be out on his own. He really has some limiting skills. I mean if you told him right now to cross the street, he might not be able to cross the street safely. He just doesn't perceive where the cars are, how to get across the street. I mean that's a 14-year-old person that can't get across the street. How is he getting anywhere? How is he going to get a car?

At the end of the interview, I asked her how she thought Thomas would be different without his autism spectrum condition. As I remember it, it was a profoundly uncomfortable moment, one in which I felt deeply aware of the intrusive impossibility of my questions—not because of any lack of graciousness on her part but because of the clarity and directness with which she struggled with all they reveal. "Oh, I don't know," she said, in response.

Maybe he wouldn't like social studies so much, so he wouldn't be as good in social studies, I don't know. That question really doesn't have an answer. I could take all the good pieces out of him and say, well if he didn't have problems socializing, and he still kept his excellent verbal skills, and he still loved history a lot, he'd be this perfect child because he has a kind heart. But what else goes away with that? So that's really hard to say. I don't really have an answer, because it's a whole person, and you're made up from all the interactions and experience you have. Whether you have a disability or not makes you who you are today. To say if you didn't have one of those interactions or experience, would you be different? Well you would be different, but you don't know exactly how you would be different.

I asked, "What about if you could go back in time, and do something to have Thomas not have Asperger's. Would you do it?"

Even more than the last, this was not an easy question. "I don't know. I don't know, you know—you know, you don't know how everything would work out if you took away pieces of it, I just don't know . . ." I could feel her sort of steel herself.

"The thing is, I definitely think it is, in fact, as Thomas says, a disease. And it is a condition. The problem is: your goal for anybody is to be a self-sufficient, thriving, person. And I think how this impairs these children is that many of them will not be able to be self-sufficient. So what services are they going to need in order to be able to live as independently as possible?"

As she remembered this—that he may not be self-sufficient, that independence requires services, that those services are often impossible to obtain in her community—she was able to come to an answer.

So if you're asking me if I'd like a cure, absolutely. Would we like to figure out how we can prevent it? Absolutely. Because the outcomes of these children, from the children that I have met, and from Thomas: how are they going to be able to be independent adults? I just don't know. Without any supportive services, I don't see it. So I would say definitely, if someone could figure out a cure or prevention, go with both, you know what I mean, because I mean how is society going to handle 1 in 150 kids?[1] I mean how do you do that? Get them to the food store, try to support them, get them medical care—all those things, I don't know, do you know what I mean? I don't know. Maybe when he passes by he looks like he's really OK, but when you get down to it, *I think he's going to need help.* I think he is. I don't know if he'll just be able to go off to college one day, you know and just go off and that's that. And not expect any help—I don't see it. You know?

Of all my interviews, the one with Thomas's mother was the one that brought home to me the nature of the dilemma in which we were embedded. Mrs. Stevenson's words stuck in my mind, and her anger in my heart, because of her refusal to deny either side of the moral conflict of cure. Amid the intense polarization of debates around a cure for autism, Mrs. Stevenson was one of few people who were able to articulate both sides of the argument—to value and cherish what Asperger's syndrome confers on those affected by it, to acknowledge the need and the vulnerability that so often comes with it as well, and then to recognize how, within the current configuration of her social world, these characteristics may not be worth their cost. She knows and appreciates her son for who he is; she believes that if he were not on the spectrum, he would not be the same person that she loves. Knowing each of these things—and not knowing how a cure would change him, only that the change would be fundamental—she would still choose a cure. She would make this choice not out of a lack of appreciation for Thomas himself—clearly not out of any lack of love for him—but because his world has no place for someone who will need help.

The sickness she sees is not only in Thomas alone but also in an underfunded school district that fights his mother every step of the way for the services to which he is legally entitled but that the district cannot afford without cutting corners elsewhere, in a medical system that went to heroic measures to save his life when he was a baby but will not address his complex medical needs as an adult, and in a job market where only the charming and compliant find consistent work. When Thomas's body was sick, the immense power of modern medicine was able to keep his heart beating and keep the air circulating through his tiny lungs until he was able to survive on his own. But these interventions on the body cannot heal him now, now that it is Thomas's social life that is sick.

The same week I interviewed Mrs. Stevenson, I sat in a meeting of local service providers, where it was announced that the state had once again cut back funding for supported housing for adults with disabilities, making it even less likely that anyone not already on the long waiting list would be able to obtain their own place to live. (There was a discussion, half-rhetorical and half-pragmatic, about which representative's office should get routed the phone calls from crying parents.) Thomas could continue to live at home with his mother, but in a culture that prizes independence above all else, the life of an adult son living at home with his parents is often seen as impoverished and shameful. And what happens when she and her husband die? There is no life story that makes sense for them. *How are they going to be independent adults without any help? I just don't see it.* Thomas's mother would choose to cure Thomas's condition not because she wants Thomas to disappear but because of the ways she fears he is already invisible.

Talking Fundamentally About What Is a Person

At the crux of intractable controversies about prevention and cure is a fundamental problem with a model of personhood abstracted from social context. Defining the self entirely as a set of individual attributes suggests that if those attributes were to be changed—even if that person still lived in the same town, born to the same family, embedded in the same network of relationships—he or she would be transformed into a different person. And those same values suggest that there would be a great loss inherent in that process, whatever else might be gained. But this ideal of the individual self as fundamentally complete unto itself, ontologically irrelevant to its extrasomatic surroundings, also leads to an undervaluation of the kind of social frameworks that render autistic lives more livable, visible, and imaginable.

One very concrete example of this process can be found in contemporary patterns of resource allocation in autism. Federal, state, and private funding directed toward autism in the United States has increased considerably in the past 15 years. However, the vast majority of these considerable expenditures are directed toward the aspects of autism that can be conceptualized and addressed within single individuals, such as basic brain science, genetics, and studies of individual behavior, leaving little left over for the kinds of social, interpersonal, and community-level interventions that contribute to a higher quality of life for people on the autism spectrum (Singh, 2015; Singh, Illes, Lazzeroni, & Hallmayer, 2009). Similar patterns have been observed in the United Kingdom (Pellicano, Dinsmore, & Charman, 2014) and Canada (Krahn & Felton, 2012). Yet, for many adults on the autism spectrum, loneliness, social isolation, and a lack of access to meaningful social roles are among the most significant problems they face (Bishop-Fitzpatrick, Mazefsky, & Eack, 2018; Hedley, Uljarević, Wilot, Richdale, & Dissanayake, 2018; Mazurek, 2013; Reed, Giles, Gavin, Carter, & Osborne, 2016).

The tendency to focus attention and resources on the problems of individual autistic bodies rather than on the social supports, job training, housing, augmented communication technologies, and other interpersonal resources that support improved quality of life among autistic people has come under increasing critique, particularly by people on the spectrum themselves (e.g., see Autistic Self-Advocacy Network, 2017; Gotham et al., 2015; Singh, 2015). In a 2010 article in *Disability Studies Quarterly*, autistic information scientist Scott Robertson observes:

> Quality of life oriented autism research has received relatively little attention when compared to the preponderance of causation oriented autism research. . . . Only a tiny fraction of scholarly articles about autism in the academic literature have examined real-life concerns presently impacting autistic adults, such as access to essential augmentative and alternative communication (AAC), social acceptance, and compatible employment options. (para. 8)

Despite these critiques, interventions to ameliorate the problems attributable to autistic difference continue be directed predominantly toward individuals, and not toward the social world where these differences, and the challenges they raise, are most manifest. This tendency to conceptualize the problems caused by autism as located entirely within circumscribed individual selves perpetuates the scarcity of supports that makes autistic particularity feel unsustainable.

Even if housing and health care were all provided to him, Thomas would still need to make his way in a world where opportunities for social inclusion and belonging, at least outside of immediate family, are selectively granted based on personal characteristics, abilities, and preferences rather than external frameworks of sustained obligation. Under conditions where self-sufficiency is a criterion for social personhood and where social relationships are won through ongoing interpersonal negotiations and the performance of a marketable identity, living with autism means living under the constant threat of social abandonment and marginalization. Outside of their families, Andrew and Trevor and Thomas will need to earn themselves a place and a social role—a job, friendships, a place in a social community—by meeting high and specific demands for which their characteristics and inclinations may not be a good fit. Within their families, they are loved and accepted into relationships of mutual responsiveness and accountability—but given the small nuclear structure of their families, that system is gone once their parents pass away. Here is the origin of the specter of the fruitcake on the bicycle that haunts Mr. Yollen, forever cycling around the periphery—fed, clothed, but still "cast away, cast out" of shared social life. The man bagging groceries at Mrs. Trent's grocery store is frightening as a harbinger of Trevor's future not because there is anything inherently wrong with bagging groceries but because Mrs. Trent knows that someone who fails to win competitive employment is seen as less of a person within her society.

As long as our identities are thought to arise solely from a combination of our particular traits and our particular history, with no attention paid to the broader networks and communities to which we belong, a cure for autism will feel like an act of violence, an erasure of such personal particularities. Yet as long as our human existence is understood to end at the edges of our skin, with no acknowledgment of our need for social life, community, and networks of mutual moral obligation and accountability that transcend individual characteristics, autism will continue to seem synonymous with social abandonment and erasure, and a cure will feel like a moral imperative. This is what the families of Brookfield helped me to understand: The conflict over cure that so sharply divides the autism community is reflective of a deeper problem within a conception of personhood presumed to end at the boundaries of the body. As long as we continue working within the same paradigm, the potential for medical intervention on neurodevelopmental differences will continue to pose an intractable ethical bind.

He Would Love It If He Had a Friend

Six years later, when I returned to Brookfield, I asked Mrs. Stevenson the same set of questions. Thomas was then enjoying his classes at the local community college and doing well at them, although he could only handle a light course load. He still wasn't able to drive and didn't feel ready to live on his own in a dorm, so he had an elaborate transportation system to get him to and from class. He looked back at his time at Valley View with great fondness; when I interviewed him, he said that attending the school was one of the best things he had ever done, crediting much of his intellectual growth to Kirk's teaching style and the safety he felt in that small community. He still didn't have any friends outside of his family but considered himself to be friends with his cousins, and he got a great deal of pleasure out of purchasing meet-and-greet opportunities with celebrities he admired.

By this time, when I asked Mrs. Stevenson if she would go back in time and make it so Thomas had never had Asperger's, she was sure of her answer.

"I would do it. Because, although he is his own unique person, *the struggles that he's had*—and he accepts it all!—but the struggles he has, he would not have had to have. So people say, you know, oh, I would keep the kid *just the way that they are*. But—and it's not that I, you know—he's a good kid. *But if I could take those struggles away*. Because he's so good mentally, he knows the struggles he has. He would *love* it if he had a friend. So I mean I certainly would like that for him. So I definitely would take it, definitely would take it away."

She looked right at me, then, and gave me a sort of crooked smile. "I dunno. Is that uncommon? Do most parents say that they would rather have their kid *just like they are*?"

I remember feeling a deep unease. "People say all *kinds* of things," I equivocated.

"It's not that you love—*I* love—him any less." She was tapping on the table for emphasis. I can still hear the rhythm on the digital recording of our interview, thrumming beneath her words. "It's that I want the best for him and to be as successful as he could be. To be the person he wants to be. And this limits that."

In this final interview with Mrs. Stevenson, I was struck by her ability to imagine what Thomas would have been like if he were not on the autism spectrum. Although many parents told me that they couldn't possibly imagine their child without autism or that they would be a different person entirely, Mrs. Stevenson was able to imagine how Thomas might still have been Thomas.

"If he was not on the spectrum, Thomas would have been—he probably would have been more similar to my daughter. I mean, physically he's muscular and he would have been broader, so he probably would have been involved in sports because my husband loves sports—we tried him in baseball and everything but it just was a disaster. I think he would have still done school, 'cause we're very much pro-school and education, so I do think he would have been at school and doing well at school."

She is able to envision her son as something more than just his traits and his history by remembering that he is also part of something broader—in this case, his family and their traditions. She considers, too, the affordances of his whole body and its potentialities for engagement in social and relational practices. Her conception of Thomas looks beyond his internal traits and attributes, taking into account aspects of personhood that extend beyond his brain into his whole body and the network of relationships and practices that surround him.

The ethics of response to the phenomenon we now call autism calls on us to reconsider not only how we think about that condition but also how we think about ourselves. In the next chapter, we will encounter resources for radically rethinking the very parameters of personhood. This alternative set of metaphors and the options they offer for a more integrated conception of autistic experience don't come from expert discourses; they don't come from textbooks or laboratories. They come from a different set of shared mythologies, emerging through the phenomenological experiences and the imaginative work of the Brookfield teens themselves.

The Sword in the Soul

Three Stories About Autism

Autism is like this.

It's like someone sneaks into your house, in the middle of the night, and takes your precious baby's mind, and personality—and leaves their bewildered body behind.
—Cure Autism Now!, "Kidnapped" (2005)

This is what we hear when you pray for a cure. This is what we know, when you tell us of your fondest hopes and dreams for us: that your greatest wish is that one day we will cease to be, and strangers you can love will move in behind our faces.
—Jim Sinclair, "Don't Mourn for Us" (1993)

This book began with these two stories about autism, dramatic in their differences. In the first, autism is a threatening invader, destructive and alien, a bearer of catastrophic loneliness and loss. In the second, autism is a constitutive aspect of the self, a source of community, identity and strength. When I began this research, the seemingly unbridgeable distance between these two stories shaped the questions I brought with me to the field. I wondered how young people growing up with autism spectrum diagnoses reconciled such divergent sets of ideas about autism, the self, the world, and the relationship between.

Over time, however, I became aware that these stories also share an uncanny similarity: Both are stories of disappearing persons. Both posit a self that is bounded and fragile, existentially vulnerable to external impingement, and obliterated if it is altered—whether by the disease or by the cure. Kidnappers steal children from their families. Strangers move in behind their faces. Nothing is left of the person that was. In these dominant autism narratives, the intrusion of that which is antithetical to the self leads to its annihilation.

As I spent time alongside the youth of Brookfield, listening to how they talked about autism, I was listening for themes I knew from these stories: self and not-self, alienation and belonging, sickness and strength, what makes us who we are and what threatens to unmake us. Before long, I started to hear these themes emerging in different kinds of stories: stories not about the mutual exclusivity of opposing elements but about their fraught coexistence. I was hearing them somewhere I hadn't expected, in stories I hadn't planned to tell. But I heard them again and again. Eventually, I started listening.

> Nightblade is a young man of about 20 who remembers nothing of his past—nothing before the day he was stabbed by his archnemesis with a sword made of pure evil. The sword did not go deep enough to steal his soul, but a shard remains embedded within him. At times, he becomes possessed by it, and transforms. In these bloodthirsty rages—his "heightened states"—he has enormous strength, and will attack even his closest friends. Even when he's not in this altered state, his eyes still glow red, and his body is mutated and twisted. He is surrounded by an aura of coldness that leads people to avoid him, though they don't know why. But deep down, his soul is still good. And though he tries to run away from his friends, to keep them safe from him, they refuse to let him go.

I had been hanging out in Roland's high school classroom at Valley View for a few weeks before he decided to show me his notebook. One day, he gave me a sidelong glance and opened the book in my direction, revealing intricate illustrations, words, rows of numbers. In this notebook, he explained to me, he spent most of each day designing a team of supernatural characters inspired by the video game Soulcalibur. Each one had their own characteristic armor and weaponry, a list of "stats" quantifying their strengths and vulnerabilities in various areas, and a "signature taunt" directed at the enemy. Each one was based on one of his friends or classmates from Valley View or the Unity Center. Nightblade, the leader of the team, was based on Roland himself.

I could see the parallels. A gangly teenager who was fascinated by medieval weapons and eager to discuss the gory details of their intended effects, Roland could be unsettling to the people around him. He had a tendency to pace to and fro while holding forth at great length about the motivations of political dictators; when upset, he burst into dark, agitated murmurs. Despite his luminous intelligence, his teachers were worried about what would happen to him if he went to college—worried that people around him would be frightened, that he might get in trouble with the police, might get kicked off campus or arrested. He is also one of the kindest people I met in my 2 years of fieldwork. But years of bullying in elementary and middle school had turned him from, as he told me, "the friendly happy person" to "a very quiet, very withdrawn, and at times very dark individual." His good soul is a side of him not everybody sees.

In many ways, Nightblade's story, too, is a story about autism. Here, however, the condition in question is neither the malevolent invader nor the vulnerable self but the relationship between. Nightblade's condition is one of uneasy accommodation of a force both alien and intimate. The incorporation of foreign elements brings him not only extraordinary abilities but also a troubled and troubling difference that drives others away and a conflicted relationship with an unnervingly multiplicitous self. Even while he benefits from his powers, Nightblade is always in tension with the energies within, always managing the risk of transformation into his darker, wilder way. But while the shard of metal within him cuts him off from the flow of normal human experience, it also brings him into fellowship with others who have been similarly altered.

Nightblade's tale is not a story of a self that disappears if it is altered, but of a self that endures, through profound discontinuities. Agonizingly compromised in his physical integrity, authenticity, and moral standing, Nightblade can nonetheless be appreciated by his friends—and by his audience—for the very tensions that have come to constitute his life story. Such a tale captures aspects of the lived experience of people diagnosed with autism that tend to be excluded from the medical models—both the model of autism as a destructive pathogen and the model of autism as value-neutral neurogenetic hardwiring—most frequently used to conceptualize it.

Autism brings both valued strengths and devastating vulnerabilities, spans the divide between the self and the surrounding world, and is experienced both as a deeply intimate element of identity and a profound disruption of it. But the most prevalent discourses about autism posit deep and irreconcilable divisions between these elements of experience. If you are a young person growing up under the description of this shifting spectrum, how do you make sense of these fault lines? How do you explain yourself? In the previous chapters, we have followed these questions through a wide variety of settings, listening to a wide variety of voices. In this final chapter, I focus on what the youth of Brookfield themselves have to say.

A Lot of It Is What I See as Myself

It's the first week of autumn, a few weeks after the end of the Summer of Adventure. There's a little chill in the air, but it's still warm enough to hang around outside. Sylvester and I are lying on the lawn outside of the Unity Center, the week before it closes for good, trying to make bows and arrows out of sticks and Scotch tape.

"Do you have autism?" he asks me out of the blue.

"Why?" I respond. "Do I seem like I do?"

"Yes," he replies impatiently, as if it ought to be obvious to me.

"How come?"

"You're fun. And you're weird. You play with swords. And you come here. And you came to my birthday party."

Once he explains his observation, it makes sense: These are the characteristics he associates with autism because these are, to him, the most interesting, important, and obvious of the characteristics he shares with other people with autism. I try to explain some of my unusual behavior by telling him that, no, I don't have autism; I am an ethnographer. So I do some similar things, but for somewhat different reasons. I've tried to explain this to him a few times, but I'm not sure it's really sticking, perhaps because the distinction between these two identities is not as relevant to him as their commonalities. Sylvester's memory is an ephemeral and fast-moving place, where things shift and change form and disappear from moment to moment. What he perceives me to be, in any given moment, is what I am for him right at that moment: a matched mind, a crafter of tools, a playmate. For the moment, I set aside my efforts and just enjoy the feeling of being included in his special club.

Like Sylvester, the majority of teenagers I spoke with had plenty to say about what they considered autism to be and how it affected their lives, but few of them recited textbook definitions or provided lists of diagnostic criteria. While they referenced material generated within broader clinical, scientific, and political discourses, their own definitions were also idiosyncratic, situated, and personal, deeply rooted in their own life experiences.

Drawing on qualitative and quantitative survey data to argue that "autistic adults should be considered autism experts and involved as partners in autism research," Gillespie-Lynch, Kapp, Brooks, Pickens, and Schwartzman (2017) observe that "autistic people often build upon unique insights derived from the lived experience of being autistic to obtain heightened knowledge about autism as a scientific construct" (para. 3). My conversations with youth on the spectrum in Brookfield corroborate this observation. But they also highlight the extent to which scientific constructions of autism fail to capture key elements of that experience, leading to the adoption of other discourses instead. Often, interviewees claimed to have forgotten whatever they may once have known about official, standardized definitions delivered through authoritative written sources. For example, when I asked Andrew Yollen what he would say if someone asked him to explain what autism or Asperger's was, he replied, "I really couldn't give them a very detailed explanation. I really don't know much, don't know much about it at all. . . . I never researched it." When I asked him again a year later if anything had happened in his life to change the way he thought about Asperger's, he replied, "To be honest, I really don't know much. I haven't really read any books about it, so I probably don't really understand what it means myself."

Despite his insistence that his lack of book learning and research on the subject meant that he didn't know much, as we continued to talk, he vividly described the practical, experiential knowledge of "how to deal with each other" that allowed him and his classmates on the autism spectrum to form a supportive community. In a mixed-disability classroom, Andrew felt lonely, left out. But at ASPIRE, and then at ASPEN, he had a different experience of his classmates.

> They knew how—they knew that: look, y'know, we have autism, we're annoying, we're hyper sometimes, we do this, we do that. So we knew each other, we got along with each other, we know how to deal with each other. . . . We all knew what it was like to be picked on and made fun of in school. We knew what it was like to be excluded, and, you know, left

out of things. 'Cause we were all different. But since we're all the different people with the same condition put together, we got along, we knew what each other was like, we never got left—we never left each other out, so we got along!

When I asked Darren how he would define Asperger's to someone who had never heard of it, he described a process of extrapolating from his own experience rather than memorizing official classifications. "That pretty much happened on the bus today," he told me. "And I was like: a lot of it is what I see from my own perspective. What I see as myself, almost."

To be sure, these interviewees provided descriptions of autism spectrum conditions well within the wide range of possibilities I had encountered elsewhere. They referenced debates about whether autism is a disease and what a cure would mean, often even before I asked about it; they described the social obstacles, focused interests, and sensory hypersensitivity that are central to clinical depictions of Asperger's; they talked about the low-functioning/high-functioning continuum and where they thought they and their classmates fell on it; they told me about the gifts and the challenges that come with a different way of thinking and perceiving the world. They talked about autism as genetic, for the most part, but often suspected that something else—lead poisoning, sickness in early childhood, some other mysterious force—had caused them to develop differently than their immediate family members. They mentioned a number of sources for all this information, including Wikipedia, YouTube videos, conversations with parents and teachers, and books they had been given or found on family bookshelves. But the way that they made use of all this material was inextricable from the specifics of their own life experiences.

Many associated autism with the traits most central to their own self-concept. For example, Trevor's social presentation relied heavily on his quirky, random sense of humor. "Everything has to be humorous with me," he told me. "If someone dies, I make it funny." Over the course of our interview, he predominantly associated Asperger's with humor and creativity: "I think Asperger's kind of helped me become creative. . . . It might have to do with how I perceive and add humor to things that I do." Darren, on the other hand, thought of himself as being highly logical. "I look for efficiency in things, you know. How they'll work best. Logical is the sense of, the science of seeing how things will work best." What he remembers most clearly about Asperger's is "the logical side—you know, more logical than social? I think that was something about it. I mean, that's one thing I've noticed and kind of relate to quite a bit."

Their experience with others who shared their diagnosis was also a factor. Trevor's banter with his classmates informed his view of Asperger's as characterized by random, creative humor; Andrew's shared experiences of social exclusion and "hyperness" informed his sense of "how we are." Timmy, a 13-year-old at Valley View, described a more frightening experience of commonality. His little brother, Stuart, was diagnosed with autism after being hospitalized with a series of seizures and a high fever and never regained the spoken language he was beginning to acquire prior to his illness. Timmy himself is diagnosed with Asperger's, and his understanding of his condition is deeply shaped by what he knows about his brother. I asked him when he first heard the term *Asperger's*, and he replied, "The second or third week when Stuart came home from the hospital. When he was fine and then—something went wrong, he wouldn't stop, like, bleeding or something? Then I go up to [the medical center], then we found out that he had Asperger's. And ever since then he hasn't talked." In fact, Stuart is not diagnosed with Asperger's but with severe autism. But Timmy has come to understand that he and his brother share the same condition, and so his conception of Asperger's is shaped by his knowledge of his brother's needs. I asked him what he thought was the best way to teach a kid with Asperger's, and he replied uncertainly: "Um, by—pictures? 'Cause that's how Stuart understands." Associating Asperger's with intellectual impairment, Timmy had been surprised to hear that Kirk, his teacher and the head of his school, had Asperger's because, as Timmy observed, "he learns like regular kids . . . he gets harder stuff really easy." According to the formal diagnostic criteria of the time, both language delay and intellectual impairment were rule-outs for a diagnosis of Asperger's; however, Timmy relied on a model that he has found closer to home.

Now That I'm With the History

These teenagers displayed a fair amount of variation in their attitudes toward a cure for autism, although most were skeptical that such a thing could be developed in a way that would affect them. Whether they would want to get rid of their autism, and whether they would rather not have had it in the first place, was largely determined by whether autism had, in their experience, facilitated or interfered with their goals and their attainment of desired roles. Luke, for example, was tenacious, kind, and very bright. His knowledge of the two World Wars was extensive; his puns were clever; his essays, which he labored over for days, were well-written, evocative, and moving. I often found myself wondering where else these gifts might have taken him had he not been so profoundly uncomfortable in so many situations, if he did not have to fight so hard to break out of routines and switch trains of thought when the situation called for it, if his need to be in constant motion—pacing, rocking, walking—did not so often interrupt his participation in coordinated group activities. Luke, too, was well aware of the ways in which his autism stood in the way of his achieving his goals, both on a day-to-day basis and in the long term. He frequently became frustrated and sad when changes in plan or unexpected obstacles shook him up so badly that he could not complete something he had started. The staff at ASPEN were working with Luke toward finding him a job in a supported employment program; he calmly, respectfully, and repeatedly noted that he would like to find a regular job.

These experiences affected Luke's views about a cure for autism, which he knew were different from that of many of his peers and the adults around him. In our interview, before I had even gotten to my questions about a cure for autism, he interrupted me politely:

LUKE: Would you mind—would you mind my views—can I say something, a bit?
ELIZABETH: Yes! Please.
LUKE: Basically, back when I was still at Unity, the people there were talking that—basically treated studies that were basically devoted to curing autism with scorn and contempt. Saying "Oh it's a condition, it's natural, you don't need to cure it . . ." I personally think that a cure should be available, but it should be an autistic person's decision to decide whether they want to be cured of it or not, if it could be researched.
ELIZABETH: What do you think a cure would do for a person with autism?

LUKE: I think that it would possibly improve their social skills, make them more like a—widen their mind, but also eliminate most of the narrowness. That's it. In other words it would basically make them back to a more neurotypical's mind. Yes.

ELIZABETH: And you think that's something that should be available to the people that want it.

LUKE: Yes.

Similarly, Richard was a history buff who had once dreamed of going into the armed forces after graduation. Now, he believed (probably rightly) that his autism spectrum disorder would prevent him from doing so. He was one of the few who said to me that, given the opportunity, he would choose to go back in time and make it so that he had never had this condition. He believed that if he could have done so, he "would have had a better future" and "would have made history" in the military rather than merely studying it. Trevor, on the other hand, wanted to become a writer. He believed that Asperger's was a determinative aspect of the way he thought and the way he viewed the world and saw it as contributing to his creativity and unique outlook. Because his autism spectrum condition was helping him achieve things that were important to him, he did not want to give it up.

Differences in symptom type and severity clearly affected the likelihood that autism spectrum conditions would hinder or facilitate one's life goals. However, these did not seem, in and of themselves, to be the major determining factors in how autism was perceived among these adolescents or whether they wanted to be rid of it. Sylvester, for example, whose behavior was far enough outside the norm that even the staff at Valley View were unsure whether he would be a good fit with their student body, valued his autism because he associated it with fun activities, events, and people. Rather, the combination of personal goals and desires, available opportunities and constraints on those opportunities, and self-perception seemed to determine attitudes toward autism among these adolescents; these factors were themselves influenced by the types of skills and impairments the students displayed.

These youth also sometimes expressed different attitudes toward autism as different aspects of their own identity became salient within our interaction. Thomas Stevenson, for example, had struggled with serious medical problems ever since his extremely premature birth: at 26 weeks, weighing 1 pound 1 ounce. His first 5 months were spent in the hospital, his childhood and adolescence crisscrossed with surgeries, intravenous tubes run through the arteries in his chest, growth hormones given to help him catch up in size, pins put in his bones to slow their growth when those hormones worked too well. From the very beginning, his development was inextricably intertwined with cutting-edge medical technology, his body shaped, for good and for ill, by new substances and interventions, along with their mysterious and often unpredictable consequences. (Mrs. Stevenson wondered if these interventions, while saving his life, may also have led him to develop autism.) From a very young age, Thomas had wanted to be a doctor. Studying medicine and medical diagnoses gave him a sense of mastery over the indignities of multiple invasive surgeries and of a body that often felt out of control. When he was talking about autism in the context of his relationship to medicine—his interest in medicine, his medical history, the medications he takes—he emphasized his struggle to maintain control of his body. "How you treat it is you just take pills for it and you try to control it, [like] you do with diabetes. You take pills and you try to control your tics or something. . . . I need them not to look like an idiot . . . doing *this* or something." He unclenched his hands from his lap and let them flap, a mannerism that he usually struggled to contain. When I asked him if he would like to be cured of autism, he told me that he would, because then he would no longer struggle with these stigmatizing behaviors.

However, Thomas's sense of his past and its relationship to his future was undergoing a shift at the time that we first got to know each other. Since starting to attend Valley View, Thomas had been studying the lives of historical figures believed by some to have been on the autism spectrum, and he had consequently gone from wanting to be a doctor to wanting to be a historian. He was already planning his first book: the autobiography of a Revolutionary War–era pirate whose antisocial behaviors, both notorious and thrilling, led Thomas to suspect he may have had autism. When he was speaking about history or his own development as a historian, he was more likely to mention the ways in which autism made people smarter and more capable:

Some famous people had autism, and look at the feats they've
achieved. . . . Because of history, I've learned to use bigger words. I've
learned facts people don't know. My family members say, "You've got
such a good memory," now that I'm with the history. . . . [If I didn't have
autism] I might be able to fit in better, but then I think I wouldn't have the
knowledge of history and the smartness I've got from that.

Just as medicine gave him knowledge of his own body and its limitations,
history has given him a sense of the previously unexplored capacities of
his mind. Each of these identities is associated with a different understanding of autism, as a bodily disability or as participation in a lineage
of troubled greatness.

Unearthing, Representing, Dividing

The youth of Brookfield are growing up at a time when developments
in psychiatric research have unearthed a condition that is multivalent,
identitarian, and worlded—what I have referred to here as the "whole
package" of autism. When I say "unearthed," I mean a process that is not
exactly creation but not quite discovery. Like an archeologist separating
fragments from the earth, the scientific practices of the neurodevelopmental turn have uncovered certain parts with certain affordances but
left others; they have chosen to focus on some parts of what emerges over
others, they have made something particular out of the parts in focus,
and in so doing, they have discovered a truth, as it has taken a form
particular to their time. This interpretive process happens through existing tools: older understandings and organizations of medicine's objects,
shaped by earlier processes of discovery made possible by other historical contexts and technologies. Medical metaphors for autism—whether
these be models of autism as a discrete disease entity, represented as
a germ, or autism as neurogenetic hardwiring, represented as a circuit—do not depict this unearthed phenomenon in its entirety. Instead,
they foreground certain elements while extruding or occluding others.

As we have seen, a model of autism as disease defines it as exclusively
negative and fundamentally separable from and antithetical to the self,
expelling the multivalent, identitarian, and worlded qualities of autism
through intertwined rhetoric and practice. The instantiations of the

hardwiring model are more complex, especially as it has been taken up by a politics of inclusion that foregrounds the varied and multiple entailments of autism and interprets it as a value-neutral difference. Here, too, however, the socially valued aspects of autism are often separated out and foregrounded—from the invocation of Bill Gates as an argument against prenatal selection to the appreciative depiction of autistic students as rule upholders. Given that these ideas are often evoked in the context of proponents justifying their own right to exist in the world, this often results in a skew toward emphasizing the particular positive contributions of autism and autistic people. Meanwhile, the sociomoral challenges posed by behavioral and interpretive difference are silenced through an association of autistic difference with a mechanized brain, while notions of "difference" are associated with value through rhetorics of diversity as an inherently desirable good.

In pointing out how socially valued attributes are often foregrounded—and morally complex challenges to social and relational networks occluded—within depictions of autism as neurogenetic identity, I do not intend to perpetuate the mistaken idea that the neurodiversity movement denies the reality of autistic struggles. Many of those working within the neurodiversity paradigm to explore its impact (e.g., see Bailin, 2019; Gillespie-Lynch et al., 2017; Kapp, Gillespie-Lynch, Sherman, & Hutman, 2013) have taken active steps to address and correct the idea that its proponents believe autism is entirely beneficial or that it brings no difficulties in need of assistance, accommodation, or sustained personal work. Instead, I want to point to the ways in which some manifestations of the neurodiversity movement, when refracted through a metaphor of neurogenetic circuitry, tend to foreground socially and economically valued qualities of autism while silencing the deep significance of autistic challenges: both the challenges autistic people themselves face and the challenges that autistic people often pose to others and to the dominant social and behavioral order.

Looking at both the model of autism as disease and the model of autism as neurogenetic hardwiring, we see that medical models predicated on the maintenance of sharply bounded individual selves within which autism is assumed to inhere cannot conceptualize the complex coexistences of the meaningful worlds with which autism is intertwined. Instead, distinctions are drawn and maintained: between mental health and developmental disability, between self and other, between that which we value and that which we reject, and between what originates outside of us and what originates within. An imaginary of the body as the bounded location point of a fragile self—a castle destroyed if it is breached, a circuit broken if it is interrupted—serves as guardian to these distinctions.

The Double-Edged Sword

For the youth of Brookfield, however, autism was inextricable from the worlds within which they experienced it; its meanings were therefore variegated in the ways that those worlds are. They tended to describe their condition as providing them with both cherished strengths and terrifying vulnerabilities; it felt both like a part of them and like something separate; it constituted their sense of self and identity while also profoundly disrupting it. Thomas, for example, defined autism to me as "a disease that affects people's understanding, and it can be very good for people, I think." These seeming opposites coexisted in complex relationships within accounts of the autism spectrum; they were not mutually exclusive but often two sides of what Roland called a "double-edged sword."

Differences in sensory perception, for example, brought benefits and drawbacks—depending on what was being sensed and under what circumstances. "The way I feel things is completely different," Roland explained to me. Sometimes this brought comfort; sometimes this brought discomfort. He could sense sudden changes in the weather, tell if it was going to rain from feeling "a sudden little raindrop that you can't even see, it's so small." He saw well in the dark but poorly in daylight. He had difficulty distinguishing between different colors. He was basically impervious to cold. He couldn't smell anything. And such a sensory difference, he vividly explained to me, could be good or not so good, depending on the circumstances:

> It's real useful when someone lets loose a real nasty fart, and holds their nose, and everyone else is choking in the room. I'll just be like, *What?* Let loose a family of full-grown skunks into the room! I'll stand and laugh, while everyone else gags and heaves! . . . But, it's also a double-edged sword in its way, as one might say. It's got its advantages and disadvan-

tages. Sure, the silent but deadly ones never affect me, nor do any of the other releases of gas in those manners. . . . But it's also a very *dangerous* thing, because I might not notice if I walk into an area with a certain dangerous odor, like someone else might walk into a room, and smell a chemical in the air, and they know it's dangerous. I could probably walk into a room filled with carbon monoxide, and never know it. I'd be *dead* before I even knew what was going wrong.

This shared difference in perspective also provided them a sense of commonality, community, and belonging with each other, even as they also experienced a great deal of social isolation and sometimes even persecution as a result of their differences. Leo, for example, described a trajectory in which alienation from the mainstream led to acceptance and a sense of community with others who were "different" in similar ways: "Aspies are estranged. They usually are alienated from the mainstream, for one reason or another. So hence they will naturally go somewhere outside of the mainstream. . . . But I believe since they are so outside of the mainstream, they go into the culture of other people who are also outside of the mainstream, because they realize, they realize 'hey, this person is not sitting with those kids too' and then those two kind of connect, for that reason."

Alienation and sociality shared a complex relationship within which these seeming opposites could transform into each other with time and changing context. When I asked how he would describe Asperger's to someone who had never heard of it, Matthew wryly replied, "I'd say it makes you really smart but you don't exactly get along well with some people." He was alluding to his long history of classroom archenemies, which he knew I knew well from my time with him at ASPEN. The impassioned, conflictual frenemy-ship with another student that made up such a central element of his time there, with its oscillating frequencies of yearning and ruptures of connection, could not be reduced to a wanted or unwanted thing. What mattered was the tension between.

It's a Part of Me, They Don't Know Where It Came From

Among all the groups and communities described in this book, a critical issue in the definition of autism spectrum conditions has been the extent to which they are separate from the affected person. "Pathogen models" of autism depict it as a discrete entity separate and separable from its host; models of autism as neurogenetic hardwiring depict it as a fundamental and determinative aspect of the autistic person, present from birth and shaping every aspect of development. In listening to the ways in which the adolescents who are the focus of this chapter talk about autism, I found that they struggled to reconcile these elements of autism using medical terminology. For them, autism felt like not only something that was part of them but also something that was separate. Darren, for example, described his condition as follows: "It's just—it's just something that's there. It's kind of like this part of me, almost. I'm not really sure how to describe it. It's a way of describing and explaining a part of me, even though it doesn't—they don't even know where it came from or how it goes around." Ever the logician, Darren became frustrated as he tried to describe something that felt both like *a part of him* and like something that *came from somewhere* else, that *goes around* outside of him as well as within him.

The medicalized theories of the body that ground popular notions of autism are closely tied, as we saw in the previous chapter, to definitions of the self as a continuously developing product of innate traits and life experience interacting over time. However, the very phenomenology of autism spectrum conditions itself poses a challenge to the notion of the human self as sharply bounded, continuous, and individually agentic. I heard this articulated most clearly in accounts of "meltdowns": intense experiences of emotional dysregulation, depersonalization, and behavioral disorganization that occur as a result of being overwhelmed with sensory or social input.

Christy, one of the Unity Center campers, was 14 when she came to the Aspie Camp. An avid reader and poet with a philosophical streak and a goofy, random sense of humor, she was always wrapped in a black velvet cloak, even in the intense July heat. This was a fashion statement, certainly, but also a way to protect herself against the sensory input that could easily overwhelm her. When there was too much going on around her, when she was swarmed or crowded by groups of people, her perceptions of the world around her disintegrated into chaos. During these episodes of psychological fragmentation, she would strike at the people around her, in a way that felt completely out of her conscious control. "I never really remember my anger things," she told me. "I remember very slightly—I remember *I was angry I hit the teacher! Oh my gosh I hit the teacher! I'm gonna get expelled!*" When I asked her if there was anything she wanted to know about Asperger's that she didn't know, she said, "Yeah—am I going to be able to, like, get a job, and live normally, and stuff?" I asked her if that was something she worried about. "Yeah. I just want a job in cartooning, but I'm afraid I'd hit somebody and they'd send me to jail." So at night, she practiced maintaining her self-control by tying herself up in bedsheets and telling herself to *stay down*.

These experiences shaped her multiplicitous sense of self. "I'm half misanthrope," she told me during our interview, laughing. "Half—part misanthrope, part creature of darkness, part anthropophobic [afraid of people]—I'm just *messed up!*" Christy's condition is inseparable from her experience of the world. It deeply shapes her perceptions, her interpretations, her interactions with those around her. But that experience is one of radical discontinuity, of deep interruptions in her sense of agency, self-awareness, and relational connectedness. Asperger's made Christy, in moments, a stranger to herself, her own worst enemy; its influence on her was often antithetical to what she saw as her best interests. Rather than interpretively cordoning it off into a disease of her body that is separate from herself, however, Christy has integrated this sense of symbiotic antagonism into her own self-concept as a paradoxically antiperson person who is "part creature of darkness."

This language of symbiotic coexistence with a malevolent force within was a not-uncommon means of resolving contradictions around the ontological status of autism. Thomas, in our discussion of a cure for autism, acknowledged that his many years of developing with the condition made it unlikely that a cure could extract it neatly from him. He did not, however, assume that autism was therefore an intrinsic, fundamental, and natural part of his makeup. Deeply steeped in the language of medicine and disease, he still imagined autism to be separate from himself, even as he also conceptualized it as inextricably bound up in his own body and history. Reaching for models to structure such a narrative, he wound up describing an antagonistic relationship with an active, quasi-agentic force within him.

THOMAS: I don't know what the cure will actually do, 'cause I've had
it for so long—most likely by the time they had one, what is it really
going to do to me? Is it a shot? Really, what is it? Because even if it's a
shot or a pill, I don't know how it's really going to affect me because
I would have had it for so many years. Maybe it'll be this thing that
they can get for babies or young kids who haven't had it for that long.

ELIZABETH: Why do you think your having had it for so many years
would make a difference?

THOMAS: I mean, like, it's so strong you can't really—do you know
what I mean? Like the pill couldn't really do anything because I've
had it for so many years.

ELIZABETH: What is it about having had it for a long time that would
make the pills—

THOMAS: It would make it immune. Like it might have developed such
power in my body it just kills the pill or something.

Thomas's hypothetical cure is a drama played out between agents that
hover between animate and inanimate: pills that can be killed, autism
that grows strong enough to do the killing, diseases that develop
immunity against human intervention. Such entities travel across the
boundaries between human and not-human, between self and not-self,
and between subject and object. Thomas is populated with quasi-objects
in the sense that Bruno Latour describes (most memorably in his 1993
book *We Have Never Been Modern*): hybrid creations that arise out of
modern projects of purification, out of the strict separation between
biology and society, nature and culture, things and beings. Such mon-
strous creatures cross established lines, combining the contents of these
circumscribed domains into entities that cannot be described, but must
be denied, by the very knowledge production systems that created them.

Thomas and Christy, Darren and Sylvester and Roland, and all the
other young people who are coming of age simultaneously *autistic*
and *with autism*, live under the description of a protean diagnosis that
shapes their status as cerebral subjects in ever-changing ways. They
experience and interpret their existence through a phenomenological
interface characterized by intensely fluctuating sensation, radical discontinuity, and a symbiotic relationship with extrasomatic materials that
blurs the distinctions between physical and cultural. They are always

already changed and changing—mutable, permeable beings, scaffolded with pins and routines, bound up in bedsheets. They are, as Trevor says, always mixing it up.

The language of medicine, with all its sharp boundaries and separations, cannot conceptualize these complex coexistences. Neither of the medicalized models of autism that circulated around these students—autism as pathogen or autism as neurogenetically hardwired identity—was able to fully capture the complexities of what it is like for these youth to live with autism: the way it brings gifts and comes with costs, the way it renders them both transgressive and productive, the way it feels both alien and intimate, the way it defines them, and the way it disrupts them. And, more important, neither one helps them make sense of how these wildly disparate elements can coexist within one person, one condition, one life. Yet the coexistence of these extremes was central to their experience of their condition. So the youth I spoke to reach for a different language, an alternative metaphorical system, a shared mythology that can better capture their relationship with their condition, with themselves, and with each other. It is a language they have gleaned not from diagnostic manuals or doctor's offices but from the pages of comic books and graphic novels. They have carried it with them from out of their hours in the virtual armor of video game avatars. It is a system of archetypes designed to be inhabited, reinvented, recombined, transformed. So they have done, and in doing so, they make sense of their own transformations.

Going Demon

Christy was one of the most devoted members of the Journeyfolk's Aspie Camp. Her appreciation for the imaginative role-playing games and fantasy quests around which the camp was structured was so great that she and her family traveled to Brookfield from several hours away, staying in a hotel during the 2 weeks of camp so that she could attend. She created the characters she would play in-game with great care, illustrating their backstories in a series of drawings. The character Christy developed to play in the final week of the game, Aura Dragonsblood, was both a mighty demon and a timid young girl. Once a gifted student of magic, Aura quit her studies so that she wouldn't become too powerful. Her greatest fear is her own anger because it allows the demon within her to take over. In such moments, she becomes extraordinarily strong, able to use her magic abilities, but she also sees the world as her enemy and can cause great destruction to those around her. Once, she even "went demon" on her best friend Victoria, leaving her friend permanently injured and reliant upon a wheelchair.

I heard these kinds of stories frequently—not only at the Aspie Camp but also woven throughout the creative work in which youth on the spectrum seemed so often to be engaged. In their art, their games, and their informal creative practices, they often imagined themselves as half-human and half-demon, pierced by shards of evil swords, or possessed by powerful ancestors—reenvisioning themselves as mutant, hybrid creatures who contained a force they struggled to manage and control. In doing so, they drew on a shared folk mythology from fantasy literature, comic books, anime, role-playing games, and other such forms of speculative culture.

These stories are often organized around moral valences in tension with one another—light and dark, good and evil—in the context of negotiating power within social relationships. *Naruto*, for example, the anime and manga series that had Sylvester so captivated, tells the story of a young ninja in training who discovers that the reason he is often mocked by fellow villagers is because he has been possessed for most of his life by a fox demon. A quirky prankster who struggles in school and is heedless of many social conventions, he is driven by a self-adopted *nindo* (or "Ninja Way") of robust commitment: He will *never* give up and *never* go back on his word. The story draws on traditional Confucian values around the maintenance of social harmony, emphasizing Naruto's individual development of particular virtues in the context of his shifting social roles and responsibilities (Born, 2009). He gradually learns to work with the power of the "nine-tails" and, in the end, becomes the village leader.

The story of Aura Dragonsblood followed a similar trajectory. In the game we played that week, the last week of the camp, villagers were being menaced by a monster who had been imprisoned years ago by a great hero but then accidentally set free. As the game progressed, we discovered that the monster was a part of the hero himself—his rage, his capacity for violence—that he had locked away, believing he needed to do so to fulfill his heroic destiny. Our quest, then, was not to destroy the monster but to find a ritual that would integrate the two sides of our divided predecessor. Within the set parameters of our game system, players had to choose between sword fighting and magic skills; however, the counselors running the game decided that as a hybrid creature (and, we discovered, a descendent of the divided hero himself), Aura could wield both weapon and wand, giving her fundamental duality a key role in both protecting her fellow adventurers and resolving the game's central dilemma.

The myths of mutant antiheroes extend the conditions they describe beyond the encapsulated brain, involving whole sensuous bodies and the worlds in which those bodies are entangled. Nightblade's transformation, for example, shifts his entire physical self-presentation—his experience both of his own body and of how his body is experienced by others. After being stabbed by the evil sword, Nightblade awakened to find one of his arms had "mutated" and become hideous. When you discover such a transformation, Roland told me, "It makes you want to get rid of whatever it is that affected you before it takes over completely." In Aura's legend, her rages change not only her body but also the bodies of the people around her: the wheelchair user Victoria, for example, whose bodily being is now entwined with the built environment and its technologies in new ways.

These stories also capture the ways in which the autism evoked in the neurodevelopmental turn transcends the individual body to run through family histories, in the form of what autistic author Dawn Prince-Hughes (2004) calls "ancestral hymns." These are the resonances between relatives that reverberate through the branches of family trees affected by genetically heritable networks of traits: An aunt's legendary eccentricities take on new meaning in light of a child's diagnosis; a grandfather recognizes and accommodates the deep meanings of a grandchild's preoccupations; a newly diagnosed adult recalls her father's desire for solitude and closely and appreciatively monitors her son's slow-growing social connections on the playground. Prince-Hughes herself tells a powerful story of how her recognition of herself in a young relative led her to feel both sympathy and intolerance for his behaviors—and eventually led her to seek out diagnoses for both of them.

The closeness of connection between family histories and autism is not adequately conceptualized in much research explicitly organized around autism as a medical-scientific concept. Ancestral hymns get written out of the stories of bounded individuals.[1] However, this theme of complex family heritability runs through the mythology of the mutant antihero. The fox demon that possesses young Naruto, for example, was placed within him by his father; woven into his struggle to learn to manage his powers is his struggle to take up his father's role. In Roland's stories, Nightblade's loyal best friend is Gravedigger, who developed "a sort of split personality" after undergoing an incomplete fusion with a powerful ancestor. In his "heightened states," he becomes incredibly intelligent but a little bit insane. "Think like Hannibal Lecter, but without the killing people," Roland told me when I asked him to explain the connection between Gravedigger's intelligence and his insanity. "He just thinks differently from everyone." That phrase—"thinking differently from everyone"—was a phrase I had also heard Roland use to describe autism. However, the broader conceptual apparatus in which autism was embedded made it less useful for these youth as a toolkit for them to conceptualize and share their experiences. Through the shared folk mythology of mutant antiheroes, these youth were able to formulate their experiences in a fuller way—and they were also more able to talk about them with each other.

Christy's best friend at the camp was Sylvester. The two became almost immediately inseparable, Sylvester tending to follow the lead of his older, taller friend as they roved together through the woods. Soon, Sylvester was playing half-demons, too. When possessed by his demon side, Feriek Ravenclaw would swing his sword wildly, rush into battle, take foolish risks, fall down in trancelike fits. "It's in my DNA," he explained to me matter-of-factly. Christy, in character as Aura Dragonsblood, stayed protectively close by him, helping him manage his transformations and minimize their destructive consequences. Midway through the game, as we walked down the path, I heard her telling him how to use meditation and favorite songs to keep the wild, angry powers from emerging and taking over—strategies that I knew she had worked hard to cultivate in her everyday life.

For all their closeness, for all they shared as youth growing up under the description of autism, for all the experiences they had in common—special schools, psychiatric confinement, ongoing psychotherapeutic involvement—I never heard these two teenagers talk together about their *symptoms* or their *coping strategies* or their *behavior plans*. When they talked to me about such things, they were shy, a bit abashed—aware of the stigmatizing baggage of these terms and practices. However, the shared folk mythology of the mutant antihero allowed them to reframe what had been a source of shame into a condition whose coexisting extremes were a source of motivation, pleasure, and meaning—both potentially generative and a little bit romantic.

The search for such congenial stories often requires autistic creators to look beyond material explicitly glossed as relevant to autism—a problem often reflected in discussions of "autistic headcanon" among fans of genre fiction. *Canon* in this context refers to the official information made available about a character or situation in the original source material; *headcanon* refers to alterations or additions to that material that fans make in their personal imaginary. *Autistic headcanon* refers to interpreting characters as autistic despite this diagnosis not having been made explicit in the source material. In a piece discussing this practice, autistic author Sarah Kurchak (2018) criticizes the ways in which characters explicitly identified as autistic in popular culture tend to hew to a certain narrow template: White, straight, cisgender men with savant skills. "Most of these characters," she writes, "appear to be constructed from the same checklist of common symptoms: no eye contact, a flat-affect voice, and generically awkward body language" (para. 6). Instead, Kurchak observes how "autistic people have been forced to get creative in our search for meaningful representation" (para. 3), claiming for themselves characters from sources such as *Star Trek* and *Supernatural*—largely, although not exclusively, speculative fiction—whose experiences of alienation, difference, and desire are rendered in richer and more diverse ways as they engage with an array of variably configured worlds (see also Queerly Autistic, 2017).

Permeable Narratives, Permeable Personhoods

These stories are a particular kind of story: Legends of permeable selves, they are themselves permeable narratives. The materials making up this shared mythology do not adhere to the kind of standards that demand great literature be canonical and complete unto itself, the product of a single and authoritative authorial voice. Instead, they are multimedia folktales, built so that readers or players can put themselves into the story and make of it what they will. Nightblade's saga was based off a video game Roland often played, slipping in and out of the bodies of its virtual avatars, shaping the events of the narrative by his own choices and reflexes. His classmates played the same game, traveled in and out of the same characters, walked the same world. The characters he created, with their list of "stats" drawn from tabletop role-playing games, were built such that they could be not only read but also actively inhabited, *played*.

Such narratives are often culturally devalued, seen as trashy and disposable, for the very reasons that make them most hospitable to their inhabitants: they privilege genre conventions, emotional intensity, and polyvocality over particularity, nuance, and individual auteurship. These kinds of texts have a long history of active use by what Jenkins (1992) describes as "textual poachers," fans who not only consume but also create and combine stories based on the fictional universes they find in popular media, mostly fantasy and science fiction. "Undaunted by traditional conceptions of literary and intellectual property," he writes, "fans raid mass culture, claiming its materials for their own use, reworking them as the basis for their own cultural creations and social interactions" in "a refusal of authorial authority" (pp. 18–19). The formulaic nature of the stories that Roland and his friends find reoccurring across video games, comic books, and Japanese anime lend themselves particularly well to this form of collective reinvention. They can be easily combined, and the familiar elements of their narratives make a comfortable space for a newcomer to join. Their consistent conventions (the tragic origin story, the banding together of misfits, the "signature taunt") not only are appealing in their thematic content but also provide a scaffold for creative expression.

In his essay "Fantasy and the Buffered Self," literary critic Alan Jacobs (2014) takes up philosopher Charles Taylor's notion of "buffered" and "porous" selves to argue that engagement with fantasy literature helps compensate for the isolation of modern self-construction. Premodern people, Taylor (2007) argues in *A Secular Age*, lived in an enchanted world in which magical forces "could cross a porous boundary and shape our lives, psychic and physical. One of the big differences between us and them is that we live with a much firmer sense of the boundary between self and other. We are 'buffered' selves. We have changed" (Taylor, 2008 para. 1, summarizing the book's argument). Porous self-hood is terrifying in its vulnerability—but in our modern, disenchanted condition, "safety is purchased at the high price of isolation" (Jacobs, 2014 para. 3). Jacobs (2014) argues that contemporary engagement with fantasy is an attempt to have a bit of the best of both worlds: "Fantasy—in books, films, television shows, and indeed in all imaginable media—is an instrument by which the late modern self strives to avail itself of the unpredictable excitements of the porous self while retaining its protective buffers" (para. 4) As our worlds become increasingly disenchanted through the growing dominance of industrial systems, fantasy as a genre plays a larger and larger cultural role. Fantasy, he argues, helps us remember how to fight back against inhuman forces and manage the consequences of our own creations. We will need these kinds of stories as we resist the mechanization of everyday life; its erasure of our subjectivity, sociality, and moral meaning; and our reduction to atomized agents.

Although Jacobs's (2014) argument is an intriguing one, it does not fully account for Taylor's (2007, 2008) observation that porous selfhood involves more than being moved by evocations of the spirit world in poetry and literature; it involves differences in the fundamental nature of the lived self-in-the-world. But people on the spectrum, whose experience of self may already be more porous than is the norm for their late modern cultural milieu, may be able to engage with this material in a way that is transformative in some of the ways that Jacobs envisions. They are not only consumers but also creators and maintainers of a mythos that holds open new possibilities for conceptualizing and inhabiting the self.

Learning from the creative work of these youth requires us to look outside of spaces and discourses explicitly constrained by medicine and its manifold histories and assumptions, delimited by procedures and paradigms that isolate and decontextualize us. For this, we need a different way of doing science: a science of the fully human and of that which exceeds humanity. Here, clinical ethnography serves us well. These ways of living under changing neurodevelopmental descriptions develop through richly symbolic, aesthetic, collaboratively co-created spaces: at the unclaimed edges of classrooms, in the pages of repurposed notebooks, in wild and temporary summer play-places, in the cracks between shifting paradigms. To see them, I needed to immerse my own self in these worlds: to hang out in Roland's classroom at Valley View, to go on sword-wielding journeys alongside Christy and Sylvester at the Aspie Camp. Responding ethically to autism requires us not to reduce it to its individual or societal dimensions but to conceptualize it in all its fullness, as it is lived and construed and manifested across its variety of enactments. Rather than drawing separations between self and other, pleasure and danger, chaos and order, power and vulnerability, the experience that gets called "autism" (and gets called many other things too) invites us to dwell in the space where they touch.

Conclusion

Bowling Together

You Can Make Something

Autism is a phenomenon that takes place at the intersection of individual and social, self and other, body and world. Where there is suffering related to autism—which is all too often the case—how can we situate interventions in that space, to mitigate that suffering? How are we to put the insights of the Brookfield teens and their creative work into practice? Within their shared, speculative mythology of mutant antiheroes, the disruptive potential of difference that straddles the edge of ordinary and extraordinary and the ever-present possibility of disorientation and discontinuity both physical and relational are incorporated within a system that imbues them with social and moral meaning. In an everyday world in which demons and magic swords hover at a periphery labeled "fiction," the thematic and structural qualities of their mythology can nonetheless offer us guidance.

In listening to people on the autism spectrum in Brookfield and Park City as they described the experiences that had been most meaningful for them and in witnessing the spaces that they created and strove to sustain, a few themes emerged. These spaces tended to be characterized by an ethic and aesthetic of connection and repair and an engagement with robust structures. They were spaces in which people came together around a shared interest or activity rather than being classified by a quantitative measure such as age or test score, allowing people to interact with (and learn from and mentor) those who might fall in different places on such scales. Implicitly or explicitly, these spaces tended to be organized around an accessible notion of virtue, one that was linked to symbolic and practical activity and thus could be cultivated through deliberate practice over time. As such, they provided opportunities for the development of moral agency and perpetuated an ethical call toward their own maintenance against the constant threat of dissolution.

A few years after I finished up my fieldwork, I went back to Brookfield. I knew that the shift from adolescence into young adulthood could be a difficult time for youth on the spectrum, and I was curious about how the youth I had known had navigated it. So I went to visit those whom I could still find, those who were still living in town and responded positively to the letter I sent around asking who wanted to do a follow-up.

Darren had struggled at first. He had started taking classes at the local community college even before graduating Valley View, but a bureaucratic mix-up had prevented him from transferring those credits into the 4-year college he hoped to attend. Meanwhile, despite being a math whiz, he kept failing college math classes; his unconventional schooling at Valley View had inspired and nurtured him, but it hadn't given him the foundations his professors expected. He got demoralized, dropped out, started working at Staples.

But a funny thing happened to Darren at the Staples: He did great. As long as he wasn't expected to work the cash register, with all its fast-paced social interaction and required sales pitches, he could contribute a lot, and his contributions were valued. "The OCD [obsessive-compulsive disorder] really helps with blocking the shelves and enjoying it!" he laughed. Some days the managers would bring him in for a shift just to tidy up the store.

Perhaps more of a surprise, he was a hit with customers on house calls. When doing computer repair, he told me, "You don't have to worry about too much else. It puts me in my comfort zone. And whatever else is compensated [for] by having this role—where I'm the guy who knows stuff. And I know I know my stuff."

But Darren didn't want to work retail forever. So he went back to the local community college, started taking classes again, and fell in love with electrical engineering. With the help of his local small business development center, he started his own independent business doing computer repair and now has a number of loyal customers. While at college, he started getting involved in clubs and organizations, such as the Phi

Beta Kappa honor society. At first, it was just for a line item on his re-sume, but he soon found he was enjoying them for their own sake. He helped to design a pumpkin-chucking catapult for the Engineering Club, gained some fame for shaving his long hair for a college fund-raiser, and then gained even more fame for designing a portable battery-powered game system that he started bringing around to campus events. "People were just begging me to come bring it anywhere I could," he told me. "I made a lot of friends that way." As a lark, he decided to run for student government, nominated by the members of the Engineering Club, and wound up liking it. He brought the portable game system to a retreat for student leaders, and it was a hit. The next year, when the cheap, unreli-able three-dimensional printer that the college had bought finally bit the dust, he convinced the Engineering Club that instead of buying a new one, they should just make their own.

This has become a bit of a mission for Darren: convincing people to make their own stuff and to learn to look after the stuff they have rather than just buying new things and throwing them away when they break. He's become a regular at monthly local community events, called Repair Cafés. He's been to every one since they started. "People come in with one or two items that need fixing. Oftentimes they're chairs, or lamps, or sweaters, or gloves, or something electronic. Toaster ovens, what-not. And get these things fixed!" The purpose of these events is "to encourage that a lot of these things don't have to be sent to landfills—and not only that, but there's local repair guys. And one of the few things you can't outsource is *local repair guys!*" He laughed. "You know? And just keep-ing these things out of landfills and just encouraging a more traditional perspective on that."

Repair Cafés assert the continued value of local coherence, even in an increasingly globalized economy of circulating, disposable goods and services. Darren is getting this "traditional perspective" from an unusual opportunity: the chance to hang out with people of a different generation. "Most of the people are much older than I am. I'm by far the youngest person who is usually there. Most people are—retired, frankly. You know? Retired, or doing whatever. It's cool, I just fit in in a weird way even though I'm half their age. I'm usually the only guy doing com-puters, a lot of times." One time he brought in that three-dimensional printer he had made himself, just to show people what can be done. "I don't have time in those 2 to 3 hours to print anything useful, but it really encourages the whole idea that: a lot of these things, you don't have to buy from elsewhere, or toss away. You can make something."

In addition to learning from those who have come before him, he also strives to be something of a mentor to younger Aspies. "I see an awful lot of kids who are Aspie—whether they realize it or not. Interestingly enough, after being at Valley View for a number of years, I've got almost this gaydar for understanding when kids have Asperger's, even if they don't realize it! Sometimes it slips out, some sort of mention here and there, just something in passing, and they'll get uncomfortable, and I realize they've heard the word, they know it's associated with them—but no one's supposed to *know!*" He laughed. "And it's like—*oops!* Y'know? And I try to pass it on, I try to encourage it, you know: *I went to a school. It's a cool thing. I've got it, I'm proud of it.*"

For Darren, the momentum of his life had started to support him in going in the direction he wanted to go. "I kind of see it as falling into a good rut, after being in bad ones. Letting myself go in the opposite direction, with good things, and just let myself keep rolling! Taking them as they come, and not worry about too much at this point. Falling into a good rut and letting myself, really, trying to keep that positive direction." The contours of Darren's life are built out of strong materials, arranged with his characteristic ingenuity and care; he is confident, competent, and content.

We Put Duct Tape on It So No One Gets Burned

When I last saw Sylvester, he had finally made it to a classroom where he could be with other kids on the spectrum, joining the younger classroom at ASPEN. "What do you think of the ASPEN program?" I asked him.

"It's great. I made a lot of friends."

"What makes the ASPEN program so great?"

"I have friends. I'm not in a normal school anymore. And I'm in an autism program, which is good. I've been waiting for that my whole entire life. Except when I didn't know I had autism."

At ASPEN, teachers worked closely with Sylvester to help him get better control over his behaviors, including putting him on a strict program where he got a time-out every time he threatened to hurt himself or anyone else. Although she was generally not a fan of behavior modification programs, Annie was proud of Sylvester for sticking with it. "I'm not just interested in having him change the behavior," she told me. "I want there to be, on the inside, the sense of mastery for him."

Sylvester felt that sense of mastery as well. When I asked him what major changes had happened in his life since I last saw him, he told me, "My major changes would be my self-control and that I'm doing an allowance thing where I get it at the end of the week. It's a really good major change for me." Practicing self-control and saving toward long-term goals had opened up for Sylvester more hope for participating in wider social worlds. "I have to say, with the self-control, that I've been actually learning self-control so I can actually rejoin the Journeyfolk. I had decided that, actually, right now, kind of was my goal because Journeyfolk was totally, like, way fun. And I really want to do the more, like, nonautistic one. So I can actually learn how they actually do it. And I want to use my dragon, elemental dragon blade, to show the competition how good I am."

In the meantime, Sylvester had taken up fencing. A local teacher had formed a group, the Fellowship of the Five Pillars, and I went with Annie and Sylvester to attend one of their tournaments. The Fellowship included a lot of quirky local kids, including Sylvester. One of the teachers told me that a few of the kids there were on the autism spectrum, but even my trained eye couldn't pick them out.

At meetings of the Fellowship, a group of adults mentor the young knights-in-training in both fencing and chivalry, codified in "codes of honor" that they design themselves. The rules are very clear—here is how you invite someone to fence with you, this is where you stand, this is the order of events at the tournament, and so forth—but at the same time, there seemed to be a lot of tolerance for noise and movement and talking out of turn. If any of it was starting to get disruptive, one of the leaders would just go *shush* and this usually worked. The youth of the Fellowship seemed very motivated to rise through the ranks: When you first start out, you can only fence with one of the instructors; then as you get better at it, you graduate to being a squire, then a page, and so on toward knighthood.

The Fellowship is an example of what James Gee (2005), a scholar of language, learning, and literacy, calls an "affinity space." Affinity spaces are defined by a set of features, of which most will share many but not necessarily all. Participants are brought together by a sense of common endeavor, which is more focal to how participants relate to each other than are each member's individual characteristics. Inexperienced newcomers and seasoned experts share common space; while they might hold different roles or classifications, these distinctions do not prevent them from freely commingling. Participants in the system may have opportunities to transform the parameters of the system itself, generating new symbolic content as well as shaping the internal grammar through which the system is governed. Affinity spaces encourage participants to cultivate knowledge that is both intensive and extensive and to both hold this knowledge individually and contribute to its shared distribution. The system honors and uses dispersed knowledge—knowledge gained outside the boundaries of the system itself—and both explicit and tacit knowledge: the knowledge that can be put into words and that which emerges instead through practice. Affinity spaces offer a variety of ways to participate, and many different routes to status; leaders are seen more as resources than as fixed roles. Such spaces offer an opportunity to cultivate social connections that are grounded in shared, meaningful interests, providing both stability and support for social innovation.

Affinity spaces such as the Fellowship support members in cultivating a sense of "moral agency" (Myers, 2015): the capacity to be a good person in such a way as to develop strong, mutual social relationships. The sociality of the Fellowship was grounded in something greater than the mere pleasure of social interaction, something larger than individual personality traits, something more solid than the transient and anxious management of bonds that exist solely for their own sake; its members were working together toward a shared notion of the good within a symbolic system that supported them in that goal. They were motivated to participate, and to care through practical action for the connections that held the group together, because they bought into that shared notion of virtue.

In this respect, the Fellowship differed significantly from the kinds of clinical groups that teach kids "social skills" as flexible, abstract concepts. Speaking from my experience as a clinical psychologist who has worked in a number of settings serving kids with social problems understood to be neurodevelopmental: A lot of the social skills groups offered to these kids are pretty grim endeavors. They often take place in hospitals, clinics, or therapy centers—not the kind of places that people tend to gravitate toward to voluntarily socialize with each other. Often, the groups get seated around a big table in some repurposed conference room, looking like a meeting of an executive board composed largely of anxious 10-year-olds. Participants are rewarded with points for refraining from talking about the things that they (and probably at least some of the people around them) are interested in—"quirky" topics like dinosaurs (too babyish) or the stock market (too grown-up). Instead, we talk about more appropriate topics—What did you do over the weekend?—that manage to be impersonal by way of being personal. Participants practice having conversations with people they know (that kid sitting next to them who they see every week, who freaks them out because he's so loud, or so quiet, or because of the way he stares, but who brings good cards to play in the waiting room) as if that kid were a generic everyperson, leaving aside any background knowledge they may have about that kid or their life or their feelings for each other. The goal is to practice a style of interaction that could be easily picked up and moved to any other person, place, or time that falls into a comparable category. After it's over, the kids can exchange the points they've been given for toys and prizes. Often, parents and/or professionals are invited to watch through a two-way mirror so that after the event is over, they can discuss with the child's therapist where they went amiss, how they could do better next time, and how parents and kids can continue this work in other areas of life—at home, in the park, around the family dinner table.

There are good reasons for doing things this way—the kids like structure; they are not thought to be intrinsically motivated to socialize with anyone, let alone with whatever random assortment of kids has been assembled for that run of the group; parents need to be involved to help the skills generalize into other settings—but it's not exactly a recipe for a good time, unless you're the type of person who likes to compete on reality shows. And it teaches a certain kind of sociality: one that is fungible, expansively commensurate, and equally applicable across contexts, to friends and strangers alike—to your customers at the McDonald's and your buddies at the bar. A kind of sociality that is organized, compelled and rewarded by external authorities, and constantly under evaluative surveillance. A kind of sociality in which interactions seem to exist for their own sake rather than for any shared purpose, but are actually serving the wishes and desires of a system that has been hidden behind the mirror. In their content, such groups may try to teach kids how to adapt social repertoires to different environments—to the classroom, to the playground, to the workplace—but in their form, they compel the occlusion of context, taking place in very particular physical and social spaces that successful participants are required to ignore rather than use or challenge.

Instead, we could support the cultivation of social settings that do not focus on rewarding compliance with decontextualized social expectations but on rewarding contributions to ongoing social projects characterized by shared, superordinate goals: not merely the pleasure of interacting for its own sake but for the purpose of building, maintaining, and participating in something larger and more lasting. "Sylvester dreams of having clubs and making clubs," Annie told me the day I went to visit the Fellowship with them. When I asked her what she thought was the most important use of resources for people on the spectrum, she replied, "Creating community—creating after-school programs that are viable, that aren't going to disappear."

"When you make a Journeyfolk blade," Sylvester told me, "you need added leverage. You can actually put duct tape on it so it creates weight on it and no one gets burned [from the roughness of the foam] anymore. That's why, in my club, we're going to put the tape on it so no one gets burned. Then we'll spray paint them so the paint—so we have colors. That's a good idea." Sylvester's dream clubs are organized around building things that aren't going to disappear: swords reinforced and strong, painted in colors, taped up such that no one gets burned.

Strength Comes in Numbers

Such community spaces are in increasingly short supply. This trend has been documented memorably by Robert Putnam (2001), whose *Bowling Alone* demonstrated a decline in American participation within sustained social spaces both within and outside the home, occurring simultaneously with the rise in private consumption of mass media, such as television. As a result, we are seeing a decline in *social capital*: the value that comes out of connections between individuals embedded in dense networks of social commitments, with benefits that accrue to both individuals and society. Americans, Putnam observes as an example, are still bowling, and watching plenty of sports on TV, but we are no longer bowling in leagues. We are bowling alone.

But I saw something very different at Jake's bowling league. Although it was a league by and for adults on the autism spectrum, Jake was very clear with me that the point of the group was not autism, it was *bowling*. (To keep my presence from making the vibe of the group too centered on a potentially pathologizing diagnostic category, I was allowed to attend only as long as I didn't just sit around talking to people about autism but actually *bowled*.) At the same time, autism provided the motivation and sense of common purpose that led Jake to keep the group going, and inspired attendees to attend. In terms of Gee's (2005) definition of an affinity space, autism became not only an individual characteristic but also a shared endeavor. "We've all had problems at one time or another with social," Jake told me. "In some cases it's very severe. That's part of the reason why I'm running the bowling group. You know, to get people out of the house and everything."

I asked Jake what kept him involved with Asperger's advocacy. "I think it's a feeling of giving back," he told me. "I mean, I've been through a lot, so I've gotten through that. I'd like to impart my experiences, trials, and tribulations of life, especially [to] these kids, most of them younger than me. Eduard reminded me so much of myself when I was younger, it's not even funny. He's very hard on himself. I noticed that he's easing up. So if I can help a person like that . . ." But Jake's goal with the group is not only to help individuals but also to help people on the spectrum band together to support each other. "Strength comes in numbers," he told me. "The very fact that we're able to have support groups with a bunch of people who are antisocial, I think it's a miracle. The fact that I have people coming to my bowling group on a regular basis, I think that's a damn miracle. I didn't think it was gonna last this long. I honestly didn't."

Spaces like the bowling group and the Repair Café are characterized by an ethic of care and maintenance of local connections—between the parts of the toaster, between the local repair guy and his neighbors, and between the craft, the craftsman, and the community—held in bonds of space-time that have not yet been dissolved. They create an opportunity to be recurrently present to each other: Think of how Doug, in his friendship with Eduard, took the same route each day to his new friend's house, in the process learning how to navigate frightening roads rather than just staying home alone.

"I would like to contribute more to the world; I really would," Jake told me. "And I think one day I will get to be that way. I'm starting to contribute over the last few years—trying to start to make my contributions." Jake feels a keen sense of urgency about his work. He is worried about his fellow Aspies, and worried about the future:

> You get the feeling that you're overwhelmed. And so if it comes too fast, too much too fast, I think it's very difficult for anyone, really, to change, very difficult. If it's too overwhelming, then that could be a problem. I think we're in for a lot of changes: the weather's been changing, climate change. There's definitely climate change going on. There's social, there's political. There's all sorts of changes going on, and the next few years is going to be too many. There's gonna be a lot of changes, and too many changes, I think, for the average person to keep up with. It's going to be very challenging to keep up. . . . And in some cases, I mean, those who can adapt to the changes will survive. Those who don't, they won't.

Cleaning Up Social Town

But the connections formed in Asperger-specific cultural spaces, and diagnostic social identity movements in general, are always at risk of being attenuated through the assumptions of the medical discourses upon which they are founded. The deep organizational structure of these medical discourses—their metaphors, their infrastructures, the presuppositions under which their stories make sense—posit a self that is sharply bounded, guarded against the outside world, easily transmuted into just another traveling game piece that can be moved between classrooms, between care providers, between social settings.

The carefully cultivated cultural practices of the Journeyfolk, the mutant mythologies of the Brookfield teens—these materials have their own internal logic, their own systems of organization that define their robustness and enact their own particular affordances. To benefit from the social capital and social healing that these spaces make possible, we must respect their deep structure and the locally coherent, stable bonds and relationships within which their meanings are instantiated. Such complex, situated systems face ongoing pressure to reduce to their surface, representational elements—those that move easily between contexts, those easily adaptable to new surroundings. We saw at the Hayes Center how easy it is for a concept to get reduced only to the elements that work within a given set of expectations, its transformative elements gradually pushed to the outside of tightly guarded doors. The result was a version of autism that evokes and then collapses the complexities of social life, rendering them newly tractable. The logic of extrusion, in which self-contained persons and societies need to be perpetually guarded against external threats, can easily make its way into and co-opt potentially transformative stories.

Superflex: A Social Thinking Superhero Curriculum (Madrigal & Winner, 2008) is a tremendously popular intervention for kids with "social cognitive" challenges, such as autism and Asperger's syndrome, that draws on the appeal of the kind of superhero mythology described in the last chapter. But Superflex is no Nightblade. A blond-haired, blue-eyed, snub-nosed fellow in a cape, with wide eyes and a big, bright smile, his job—and the job of kids training the "superhero in their brain" at the "Superflex Academy"—is to defend the inhabitants of Social Town from the team of "Unthinkables" that stand in the way of Social Thinking. "While Superflex has powers to provide people with flexible thinking and problem-solving skills" reads the introductory material, "the Unthinkables have the power to derail specific aspects of social behavior, leading us to do something unexpected" (Winner, 2018, para. 4). The Unthinkables, drawn as vivid anthropomorphic cartoon figures, cause unexpected behavior by afflicting their victims with various forms of inflexibility. Rock Brain makes people rule-bound and rigid; Topic Twister Meister makes people change the subject to things they are interested in rather than what others are interested in. Glass Man does not bend but shatters, getting upset over problems others think are unimportant. He gets especially upset, the worksheets tell us, over things that seem "unfair" (scare quotes in original). There are many more Unthinkables; a contest asking kids to suggest their own Unthinkables drew hundreds of entries (Winner, 2015).

To defeat the Unthinkables, Superflex uses a series of strategies. For example, one way to defeat Rock Brain when among others is to "ask yourself, 'What is their plan?' And then try to match their plan" (Madrigal & Winner, 2008, p. 86) The end goal is to create a brain/society that is free from problematically idiosyncratic obduracy. One of the early assignments in the Superflex Curriculum is called "Cleaning up Social Town." The instructions read: "The Unthinkables have all been defeated!!! Create a picture of what Social Town would look like now. Draw three examples of citizens using their Superflexible thinking and thinking about others. Ahhhh . . . What a great place to live" (Madrigal & Winner, 2008, p. 26).

With its talk of superpowers, adversaries, and brains pervaded by imaginary characters, Superflex draws on the mutant mythos that youth on the autism spectrum often use as a way of reconciling aspects of their condition and restoring its moral meaning. (Similarly, Winner and her team—see Winner & Crook, 2011—have also created a program for teens, called Social Fortune or Social Fate, that is drawn in the manga style of Japanese anime. Rather than highlighting Confucian cultivation of virtue in the context of social relationships, as manga such as *Naruto* do, however, it revolves around the idea that individual actions determine one's social place, teaching teens to use strategies such as "Think About Choices" and "Minimize a Reaction to a Problem.") In the case of Superflex, however, this mythology has been changed from a story of inclusion to a story of extrusion. The potential for extremes of emotion, experiential shattering, a failure to flex, an unwillingness to "match the plan" is not incorporated but instead banished from the metaphorical body-polis. Resistance is rendered Unthinkable.

From the very days when Hans Asperger first made his observations of his "little professors" under the watchful eye of the Nazi regime, the articulation of these neurodevelopmental differences has been organized around the separation of valued from devalued difference, and the protection of the former at the cost of the banishment of the latter from our concept of the human. Many of the stories currently flourishing within medical systems are organized around such strict borders and boundaries, these logics of separation and exclusion. Sociologist Zygmunt Bauman (2000) believes that the body "has become the last shelter and sanctuary of continuity and duration" (p. 184) in a time of fluidity and flux. "The boundary between the body and the world outside," he notes, "is among the most vigilantly policed of contemporary frontiers" (p. 184). This vigilance around the boundaries of the body serves as a metaphorical model for society: what belongs within and what needs to stay outside. He observes

> the tendency to shape the image of community (the community of certainty-cum-security dreams, the community as the greenhouse of safety) after the pattern of the ideally protected body: to visualize it as an entity homogeneous and harmonious on the inside, thoroughly cleansed of all foreign, ingestion-resistant substances, all points of entry closely watched, controlled and guarded, but heavily armed on the outside and encased in impenetrable armour. . . . The body and the postulated community alike are velvety on the inside and prickly and thorny on the outside. (p. 184)

But other stories take place in other spaces—stories of permeation, of openness to the environment, of painful, confusing, and generative co-existence. Other possibilities can grow in settings that include both the velvet and the thorns, honoring the connections and tensions between them. In such places, we can hold and be held by the structures of things in the world as they are—and we can dream of what else they could be. Our armor is breached, and new worlds appear.

Ad Astra, per Aspera

I met Phillip at a science-fiction convention. I had gone there to hold a series of focus groups about Asperger's syndrome and sci-fi fan culture. When I announced to the lobby full of convention attendees that I was planning to hold a discussion on Asperger's, Phillip sat down next to me and declared, "Oh yes, I've been diagnosed with that." (People had told me that this sort of thing was likely to happen at science-fiction conventions, which is why I was there in the first place.)

Phillip, too, had a particular purpose in coming to the event. "I came here out of the blue—literally, in fact, in an airliner, a distance of over 2,000 miles—specifically for the reason of finding people who were interested in the project of settling the moon." Neatly attired in a three-piece suit and felt hat, precise in his diction, and formal in his language, Phillip looked and sounded like someone from an earlier century. But he had his eyes firmly set on the future. "I would assert that space development is something which is necessary for the happiness and continued survival of the human race in the coming few hundred years, possibly in the coming few decades. We need new sources of metal. We need new sources of energy. We need what space can give us, in material terms. As long as we're locked into the earth's resource base, we're going to have serious problems. And of course the doomsday argument is that there are half a dozen causes which could cause the extinction of life on earth in the next 100 years." He smiled wryly. "Some might debate whether it's a *good* thing for humans to survive—but I think that a lot of us would feel it was better for the human race to survive than not to survive."

Since dropping out of college due to stress headaches and ill health, Phillip has devoted himself full-time to the project of citizen-driven lunar settlement. "I can say with confidence that NASA [National Aeronautics and Space Administration] won't do it, so we can simply ignore them. They've had 35 years since Apollo 17. If they were going to give us the stars, we would have had them by now. So we can just count NASA out of the equation. Similarly, the big industrial firms, and to a great extent the small industrial startups, have the problem that they simply can't raise the capital and sink it on something without an immediate return. This is why I am looking for a cooperative; a subscription model if you will; an open-source development model." He spends most of his time traveling between conferences and conventions, giving talks, and recruiting collaborators: engineers, donors, project managers, a publicity team. "In a certain sense, anything you can think of to do is useful. I tell people: You're a musician? All right. If you're out on the street with a hat and a little sign that says: *half the money you give me tonight goes to send a man to the moon*, that's good! Especially if you actually take half that money and send it to us . . ."

Phillip didn't think of himself as having a disorder:

I think the word *syndrome*, the pathological connotations, is really inaccurate. I mean, OK, maybe I have traded, in my brain, a big chunk of the area which does nonverbal communication for the ability to work partial differential equations. Honestly I think that's a fair trade. A certain percentage of the population cannot work indefinite integrals. I can. I'm not sorry with the trade. I'm not sorry about it at all. And what I would like to see, actually, is an acceptance that people like me have a definite function in society; that we're not flawed. The fact that we don't behave the way that so-called *normal* people do is an asset to society rather than a danger.

Yet Phillip's style of interacting with the world has not been easy, for himself or for those around him:

I am a lot closer to what you'd call the *normal,* I guess, in my reactions and my behavior than I once was. Even my parents found it very difficult to communicate with me, very difficult to deal with me when I was small. In school I was what they called a *behavioral problem.* I didn't get along. I got in fights. I'm not a fighter, I don't enjoy violence, but apparently there were people who liked to beat me up. I tend to do what I'm going to do, and if it isn't what you want, maybe you should adjust your expectations. Which doesn't always endear me to people, but on the other hand, I've discovered over the years that I have difficulty endearing myself to people *all* the time.

Consequently, his life has been a lonely one, although at first, he tried to downplay this. "You could say that part of my early thoughts about space travel was just to get away—but it's not really like that. Partly it's just wanderlust. I come from a peripatetic family. My grandfather, who just died at the age of 94, had a terminal case of foot itch, and horizon fever. He was always moving. If he didn't move his house once in five years you knew he was seriously ill." Space travel, in Phillip's view, provides humanity not only access to material resources but also an outlet for such wanderers, a "psychological safety valve, as a human race. A way for people to get out, if they feel a need to get out."

But as Phillip and I kept talking, I started to get a feeling for how his alienation on earth was driving him toward the stars.

To be perfectly honest—some of my thoughts about getting out of the earth or whatever were originally motivated by a feeling of wanting to start over again somewhere else. I don't try to fit in, because I tried it, a lot, when I was younger, and it just didn't work! And after a while I give up doing things that don't work. They say insanity can be defined as doing the same thing over and over again, despite the fact that it doesn't work. That's one thing that I don't do. After the 12th or 120th time, I typically move on to pastures new.

And Phillip's new pasture might be a lonely place indeed, cold and airless, dazzled with radiation. One of the challenges of space travel, he told me, was loading a rocket ship with enough fuel to get to the Moon and back. With no planned return trip, a lunar traveler would be able to carry a great deal more resources for settlement. As we were standing together waiting for the elevator, Phillip told me that he was willing to be the first to go. He was willing to undertake this journey as a one-way mission. And he was willing to go alone.

Phillip wants to go to the moon for the good of humanity. But he also wants to go because he senses that there is no place for him here: no remaining frontiers for him to push against, no meaningful work for his kind of mind, and no company for his kind of heart. I feel for his loneliness and alienation; I admire his bravery; above all, I respect his capacity to expand the bounds of the thinkable. The world is better off with people like Phillip: weird, dogged misfits; people who come up with crazy ideas and pursue them with inflexible, unswerving determination; people willing to go that extra mile (or 2,000 miles) for what they believe even if the cost to their own happiness and comfort is high. Phillip's gift is not merely his potential for technological innovation, not merely the possibility that he will build new and better machines for us but also the possibility that he will catalyze new modes of creative collaboration toward a common goal. Phillip's power lies not only in his capacity to work indefinite integrals but also in the loss he believes he has sustained in trade for it. His inability to stay comfortably put within the confines of his social surroundings drives him to push constantly at the edges of the conceivable world, seeking to transcend its bounds. But the moon, despite his best efforts, is still very far away. There needs to be a place for Phillip here on Earth.

ACKNOWLEDGMENTS

Where do I start? I couldn't even tell you when I began working on this book. Maybe it started when I was 6 years old, spending a fun few days playing games, answering questions for appreciatively attentive adults, and getting wires glued to my head. Only later did I understand that this was a neuropsychological evaluation, aiming to make sense of the way I could read books for seventh graders but couldn't catch a ball. Or maybe this book started at Swarthmore College, when I was an undergraduate, sitting astonished in psychology seminars with Jeanne Marecek and Ken Gergen. They were the first to show me that I could take seriously as a scholar the stories and symbols that my goth posse of friends and I took seriously in our everyday lives. At the end of my time at Swarthmore, Jaqueline Mattis, my external examiner in the Honors program, gave an exam so thought-provoking that I was certain I was going to fail it. Instead, she suggested I pursue a career in the field of psychology. Much of what followed is beholden to that one moment.

Like many books of this sort, this volume began to take form in earnest during my graduate school years, which means it is, among other things, a book about what it is like to be a graduate student. I had the good fortune to be a graduate student at the University of Chicago, at what was then known as the Committee on Human Development (now the Department of Comparative Human Development, or HD for short). Tanya Luhrmann's mentorship has been a great gift; the courage and clarity of her scholarship are inspiring. Richard Taub, Eugene Raikhel, John Lucy, Sydney Hans, Bert Cohler, and Don Kulick provided inspiration, thoughtful guidance, and a Chicagoan lack of tolerance for the inadequately executed that has served me in (more or less) good stead ever since. Outside the Department, Kathryn Beth Angell and Morris Fred provided counsel both welcoming and wise. I don't think I've ever felt as happy and comfortable amongst a group of people as I did with my fellow graduate students in HD. Bambi Chapin has always been a firelight, drawing friends and colleagues together around her warmth and illumination. Mike Kaufman kept many wheels turning. From the writing group I shared with Lara Braff, Amy Cooper, Pinky Hota, Christine El Ouardani, and Ben Smith, I learned not only about my own writing and about their fascinating topics (*that thing about marbles and alpaca!!*) but also about how to give and receive feedback in a community. Kathryn Goldfarb, Hallie Kushner, Neely Laurenzo Myers, Nicole Martinez-Martin, Kim Walters, and Talia Weiner also offered good thinking and good friendship that contributed to this book. From ill-advised pitchers of beer at the Cove to jamming at the piano with each other's kids, I have cherished our times together, and I hope for more to come. Taking a small seminar with Ian Hacking on the topic of Making Up People was an extraordinary opportunity to work through many of the ideas contained in this book with a bright and like-minded group of folks. The Council on Advanced Studies workshops at Chicago were a joy and a good kind of challenge. Without the Clinical Ethnography workshop, and the workshop that had many names but that I remember best as "Culture, Life Course, and Mental Health," this book would be something very different and not nearly so interesting.

The research on which this book is based was made possible by financial support from several sources: a National Institute of Mental Health Ruth L. Kirschstein National Research Service Award, a National Science Foundation Dissertation Improvement Grant through the Science and Society program, and a Dissertation Fieldwork Grant from the Wenner-Gren Foundation for Research in Anthropology. Thanks to all these organizations for their faith in, and support of, my work and my training.

I am particularly fortunate to have been welcomed into the community of psychology faculty and students at Duquesne University. Since its early days, the Duquesne Psychology Department has been dedicated to exploring the question of how to take up psychology as a particularly human science. My colleagues there are a delight—warm and thoughtful and fun. Special thanks are due to Leswin Laubscher and Jim Swindal, both of whom fought to protect space and time for me to write this book. The writing process itself was supported over several summers by the Wimmer Family Foundation, a vital resource for junior faculty at Duquesne. Much writing, along with coffee consumption and collegiality, also took place at the retreats offered by Duquesne's Center for Community Engaged Teaching and Research.

As I try to figure out what it means for me to be a psychologist, the Society for Qualitative Inquiry in Psychology, a section of the American Psychological Association's Division of Quantitative and Qualitative Methods, has provided an intellectual home both cozy and revolutionary. (Want to join? Find us at sqip.org.) That project has also been nurtured by my fellow members of the Pizza Illuminati, and by the graduate students I have supervised on their own research who have had patience with my constantly asking them, "How are you doing psychology?"

Many of the ideas in this book flourished in the company of the participants in "Autism in Global, Local and Personal Perspective: A Cross-Cultural Workshop," held at the State University of Rio de Janeiro in September 2015. Special thanks are due to my co-organizer, Clarice Rios, the kind of collaborator who works comfortably and effectively in the realms of both grand ideas and small details, and to the Lemelson/Society for Psychological Anthropology Conference Fund, made possible by a generous donation from the Robert Lemelson Foundation, for funding the event.

Throughout the writing process, I have received thoughtful commentary from a number of scholars whom I deeply respect. Eileen Anderson-Fye, Michael Bakan, Joseph Calabrese, Marjorie Faulstich Orellana, Roy Richard Grinker, Kathryn Goldfarb, Doug Hollan, Janice Jenkins, Hallie Kushner, Rebecca Lester, Joe Masco, Jonathan Metzl, Michael Orsini, Martyn Pickersgill, Dawn Prince-Hughes, Abigail Rosenthal, Chloe Silverman, Jason Throop, Ira Van Keulen, and Matthew Wolf-Meyer have all provided insights, comments, and perspectives on various pieces of this work. I am grateful to Elinor Ochs, and to Olga Solomon for inspiring work as well as good friendship. Barbara Andersen has the kind of clear mind and listening heart that I aspire to in my own scholarship, and I am grateful to have had her apply both to the entirety of the manuscript. Christine El Ouardani, thanks for sharing the ups and downs of the book-writing process. Given that the nature of a space fundamentally shapes what happens within it, I'd like to acknowledge both Bantha Tea Bar and Lili/Kaibur Café, where a great deal of this book was written.

Participating in the Anthropologies of American Medicine series at NYU Press has been good for me and good for this book. The four external reviewers who gave feedback on this manuscript in various stages did so with remarkable generosity, perspicacity, and care. Paul Brodwin's vision of what this book can do helped me to figure out how to actually do it. Jennifer Hammer has been a thoughtful and responsive editor, helping me navigate the many branching pathways through the tangled forest of book writing. Thanks also to Martin Coleman, with whom I have enjoyed many conversations about the nuances of language and punctuation throughout the production process.

For keeping my life filled with music, thanks to Reuben Surrender, Michael Verzani, Elysabeth Grant, and Brian Allemana; James Taintor; Mathew Fuller; Manny Thiener and everyone at Treasure; and Leslie Chabala, Jessie Farine, Thomas Jenkins, and Jonathan Aryeh Wayne. I've learned a lot about role-playing games from conversations and collaborations with Erik Parsons, Chris Day, and the game writers of Peaky Midwest. Thanks as always to Ryan Woodworth, muse and arcade-game adventurer. From my parents, Scott Nickrenz and Paula Robison, I learned firsthand about how creativity, love, and community help strange children flourish. Thank you for raising me right. The past few years have involved not only writing a book but also building a home; through the whole process, my husband Peter Fein has kept me well-fed, laughing, and loved. Thank you for your Pete-ness.

It's strange to be writing this whole section full of names, Important Names of Important People, when I can't say the names of the most important people of all: the people who participated in my research by allowing me to become a watchful part of their lives and by helping me to find a place in their communities. You let me in when I was lost. You let me hang with your family and sword fight in your backyard. You shared your tangerine soda. You told me the truth. You talked to me even though you weren't sure you trusted me, because you thought what I was doing was important. You told me to turn the tape recorder off when you wanted it off. You told me I was leaning too close. You showed me how to use kitty litter to get my car out of the ice. You gave me a ride. You gave me a silver stone. You let me help, even after I screwed it up. You showed me your house. You showed me your test results. You showed me your comics. You showed me my answers, to the questions that drove my project. Thank you.

This book is dedicated to everyone out there whose ways of perceiving, processing, interpreting, learning, and remembering the world differ in some significant way from the expectations of the people around them. With this dedication, I seek to honor the creative work that you are doing, every day in many different ways, to dream a different world into being.

NOTES

INTRODUCTION

1 Exceptions include the work of Nancy Bagatell (2007, 2010) in the United States and the work of M. Ariel Cascio (2017) in Italy.

2 I have removed illustrative examples from these criteria for the sake of brevity; the full criteria can be found at www.cdc.gov/ncbddd/autism/hcp-dsm.html.

3 It is in this sense that Gil Herdt (1999) first coined the term for his studies of sexual cultures, in Papua New Guinea and Chicago. His use of the term *clinical* was inspired by the relevance of psychoanalysis to the search for a deeper psychological understanding of human sexual behaviors and their embedding in shared cultural meaning-making systems. Herdt defines "clinical ethnography" as "the intensive study of subjectivity in cultural context" further specifying that "what distinguishes clinical ethnography from anthropological ethnography in general is (a) the application of disciplined clinical training to anthropological problems, and (b) developmental concerns with desires and meanings as they are distributed culturally within groups and across the course of life" (Herdt, 1999, p. 106). The desire Herdt evokes has lain somewhat latent ever since. Calabrese (2013), for example, defines clinical ethnography as "a research approach that seeks to combine and balance the anthropological method of participant observation with clinical understanding and evaluation of self and others, derived from years of clinical training and practice" and as "culturally and clinically informed self-reflective immersion in local worlds of suffering, healing, and well-being to produce data that are of clinical, as well as anthropological, value" (pp. 51–52).

4 The Y2K bug was a problem in some computer code written in the 20th century that abbreviated years to two digits (i.e., "98" for "1998"). Many of those familiar with the problem were concerned that systems using such code would fail simultaneously in unexpected ways once their dates became incorrect with the start of the new millennium (the Year 2K, or 2000), with unpredictable and potentially destabilizing effects on technology, industrialization, and society as a whole. Due, in part, to a concerted collective effort to repair affected systems, this crisis did not come to pass.

5 Although the Centers for Disease Control and Prevention reports autism rates in the United States at 1 in 59, the World Health Organization (WHO, 2018) estimates worldwide prevalence at 1 in 160 children; the WHO (2018) online Fact Sheet on autism spectrum disorders observes that "reported prevalence varies

substantially across studies." However, "the prevalence of ASD [autism spectrum disorder] appears to be increasing globally" (WHO, 2018, para. 4–5). The particular forms that the diagnosis of autism takes in the present moment, has taken in the past, and will take in the future are clearly deeply contingent upon the historical, social, and political circumstances that produced them.

CHAPTER 1. THE SUMMER OF ADVENTURE

1 This chapter draws on material previously published in Fein, E. (2015). Making meaningful worlds: role-playing subcultures and the autism spectrum. *Culture, Medicine, and Psychiatry, 39,* 299–321.

2 What a tidy project! Alas for plans.

3 Thanks to Matthew Calhoun (personal communication) for bringing this connection to my attention.

4 There is no shortage of research suggesting that people with autism spectrum diagnoses often don't do the things in their stories that a good story, according to the researchers, is supposed to do. Their autobiographical narratives, in particular, have often been found lacking: vague and repetitive rather than specific as to time and place, not organized around a structure of high point and resolution, containing only a limited number of evaluations of their own mental states and the mental states of others (see Brezis, 2015, for a comprehensive review). In one study, they gave more detailed recountings of stories from a storybook than from their own lives (Losh & Capps, 2003). According to a theory of narrative that privileges stories specific to time and place, grounded in the unique experience of the speaker, organized around a high point and resolution, and rich with detail about internal states, autistic narratives are consistently found lacking. However, taking these findings to suggest that people on the autism spectrum are somehow *unstoried* requires overlooking the profound role of narrative, of one kind or another, in many autistic lives—and forecloses the space this narrativity opens to consider a wider sense of what a story can be.

5 Imogen was the first to make me aware of the significance of this developmental progression. One day when she saw I was having a hard time managing all my roles, she sagely observed that I was in the strange position of having to play SPCs without ever having played PCs.

6 The situation resembled Rebecca Lester's (2011) experience in an eating disorders program, struggling to translate a teenager's auspiciously rebellious choice to wear black nail polish into the standardized outcome measures dictated under managed care.

7 Andrew, unfortunately, was sick that day.

CHAPTER 2. SEARCHING FOR A PLACE

1 For example, Understood.org, a website put together by the National Center for Learning Disabilities in collaboration with fourteen other nonprofits to provide information for parents of children with learning disabilities, states that "IDEA

says that children who receive special education should learn in the least restrictive environment. This means they should spend as much time as possible with peers who do not receive special education" (understood.org, n.d., para. 3).

CHAPTER 3. INNOCENT MACHINES
1 This chapter and Chapter 4 draw on material previously published in Fein, E. (2011). Innocent machines: Asperger's Syndrome and the neurostructural self. In I. van Keulen & Martyn Pickersgill (Eds.) *Sociological reflections on the neurosciences* (pp. 27–49). Bingley, UK: Emerald Group Publishing Limited.

CHAPTER 4. HARDWIRED
1 While pointing out the pervasiveness of this distinction, in both online and face-to-face communities I encountered in the course of my fieldwork, I also want to recognize the work of scholars and activists who are actively working instead to build solidarity between these groups. For example, in April 2018, autistic writer and disability advocate Lydia X. Z. Brown offered a webinar through the Icarus Project on "Movement Work at the Intersections of Neurodiversity, Mad Pride, and Disability Justice"; similarly, the blog "Intersectional Neurodiversity," run by self-identified "neurodivergent academic" Robert Chapman (n.d.), takes as its focus "how the struggles of autistic persons intersect with other neurodivergent categories, and, in turn, with other disabled, excluded, oppressed groups, globally" (par. 2; see also Antonetta, 2007; Graby, 2015; McWade, Milton, & Beresford, 2015). That said, these efforts are working against numerous structural and institutional forces that entrench distinctions between these conceptual entities. In the communities I studied, much less was made of the points of solidarity between psychiatric disorder and neurodiversity, and much more was made of the radically new and different affordances of autism—some of which, I argue in Chapter 5, relates to novel aspects of the fundamental structure of the diagnostic category itself.
2 Cure Autism Now is a large autism advocacy organization; it has now merged with several other organizations to become Autism Speaks.

CHAPTER 5. THE PATHOGEN AND THE PACKAGE
1 This chapter draws on material previously published in Fein, E. (2016). Our circuits, ourselves: What the autism spectrum can tell us about the Research Domain Criteria Project (RDoC) and the neurogenetic transformation of diagnosis. *BioSocieties, 11*, 175–198.
2 This history is drawn from Mayes and Horowitz (2005), Luhrmann (2000), and Spiegel (2005).

CHAPTER 6. THE DIVISION OF A SYNDROME
1 She is drawing the term *malemployment* from Mark Romoser (2000), a scholar and community advocate on the autism spectrum who defines malemployent as

"working not only far below your skill level but also at a task for which you are totally unsuited" (p. 246).

CHAPTER 7. THE DILEMMA OF CURE

1 The estimated prevalence rate of autism spectrum disorders among children in the United States at the time I conducted this interview was 1 in 150 (see Centers for Disease Control and Prevention, 2019, for a historical summary of rates over time).

CHAPTER 8. THE SWORD IN THE SOUL

1 For example, see Anderson, Roux, Kuo, and Shattuck (2018) for a scoping review that demonstrates the striking absence of such social-ecological factors in the majority of autism research, despite their demonstrated causal influence on a number of outcomes.

REFERENCES

Abi-Rached, J. & Rose, N. (2010). The birth of the neuromolecular gaze. *History of the Human Sciences*, 23(1), 11–36.

alice-royal. (2015, July 20). Mental illness vs. autism/neurodiversity [Blog post]. *Little Treasures*. Available at http://alice-royal.tumblr.com

American Psychiatric Association. (1968). *Diagnostic and statistical manual of mental disorders* (2nd ed.). Washington, DC: American Psychiatric Association.

American Psychiatric Association. (1980). *Diagnostic and statistical manual of mental disorders* (3rd ed.). Washington, DC: American Psychiatric Association.

American Psychiatric Association. (1994). *Diagnostic and statistical manual of mental disorders* (4th ed.). Washington, DC: American Psychiatric Association.

American Psychiatric Association. (2013). *Diagnostic and statistical manual of mental disorders* (5th ed.). Arlington, VA: American Psychiatric Association.

Anderson, K. A., Roux, A. M., Kuo, A., & Shattuck, P. T. (2018). Social-ecological correlates in adult autism outcome studies: A scoping review. *Pediatrics*, 141(Suppl. 4), S306–S317.

Andreasen, N. (2001). *Brave new brain: Conquering mental illness in the era of the genome*. New York, NY: Oxford University Press.

Antonetta, S. (2007). *A mind apart: Travels in a neurodiverse world*. New York, NY: Penguin.

Asperger, H. (1991). "Autistic psychopathy" in childhood. In U. Frith (Ed.), *Autism and Asperger syndrome* (pp. 37–92). Cambridge, England: Cambridge University Press. (Original work published 1947)

Attwood, T. (1997). *Asperger's syndrome: A guide for parents and professionals*. London, England: Jessica Kingsley Press.

Attwood, T. (2002). *Asperger's syndrome: A guide for parents and professionals with Dr. Tony Attwood* [DVD]. United States: Future Horizons, Inc.

Autistic Self-Advocacy Network (2017). Before you contribute to Autism Speaks, consider the facts. Available at https://autisticadvocacy.org

Avery, J. (2020). *An ethnography of severe intellectual disability: Becoming "dirty little freaks."* London, England: Palgrave Macmillan.

Bagatell, N. (2007). Orchestrating voices: Autism, identity and the power of discourse. *Disability & Society*, 22, 413–426.

Bagatell, N. (2010). From cure to community: transforming notions of autism. *Ethos*, 38, 33–55.

Bailin, A. (2019, June 6). Clearing up some misconceptions about neurodiversity [Blog post]. *Scientific American: Observations*. Available at https://blogs.scientificamerican.com

Baio, J., Wiggins, L., Christensen, D. L., Maenner, M. J., Daniels, J., Warren, Z., . . . Dowling, N. F. (2018). Prevalence of autism spectrum disorder among children aged 8 years—Autism and developmental disabilities monitoring network, 11 sites, United States, 2014. *MMWR Surveillance Summaries*, 67(6), 1–23.

Bakan, M. B. (2014). Ethnomusicological perspectives on autism, neurodiversity, and music therapy. *Voices: A World Forum for Music Therapy*, 14(3). https://doi.org/10.15845/voices.v14i3.799

Bakan, M. B. (2018). *Speaking for ourselves: Conversations on life, music, and autism*. Oxford, England: Oxford University Press.

Banich, M. T. (2009). Executive function: the search for an integrated account. *Current Directions in Psychological Science*, 18, 89–94.

Baranek, G. T. (2002). Efficacy of sensory and motor interventions for children with autism. *Journal of Autism and Developmental Disorders*, 32, 397–422.

Baranek, G. T., David, F. J., Poe, M. D., Stone, W. L., & Watson, L. R. (2006). Sensory Experiences Questionnaire: Discriminating sensory features in young children with autism, developmental delays, and typical development. *Journal of Child Psychology and Psychiatry*, 47, 591–601.

Baron-Cohen, S. (1995). *Mindblindness: An essay on autism and theory of mind*. Cambridge, MA: MIT Press.

Baron-Cohen, S. (2000). Is Asperger syndrome/high-functioning autism necessarily a disability? *Development and Psychopathology*, 12, 489–500.

Baron-Cohen, S., Richler, J., Bisarya, D., Gurunathan, N., & Wheelwright, S. (2003). The systemizing quotient: An investigation of adults with Asperger syndrome or high-functioning autism, and normal sex differences. *Philosophical Transactions: Biological Sciences*, 358(1430), 361–374.

Baron-Cohen, S., Wheelwright, S., Skinner, R., Martin, J., & Clubley, E. (2001). The Autism-Spectrum Quotient (AQ): Evidence from Asperger syndrome/high-functioning autism, males and females, scientists and mathematicians. *Journal of Autism and Developmental Disorders*, 31, 5–17.

Bascom, J. (Ed.). (2012). *Loud hands: Autistic people, speaking*. Washington, DC: Autistic Self Advocacy Network.

Bassiri, N. (2016) Plastic reason: An anthropology of brain science in embryogenetic terms (review) [Blog post]. *Somatosphere*. Available at http://somatosphere.net

Bauman, Z. (2000). *Liquid modernity*. Cambridge, England: Polity Press.

Beck, U. (2002). The ambivalent social structure: Poverty and wealth in a 'self-driven culture.' In U. Beck & E. Beck-Gernsheim (Eds.), *Individualization: Institutionalized individualism and its social and political consequences* (pp. 42–53). London, England: Sage.

Beck, U., & Beck-Gernsheim, E. (2002). *Individualization: Institutionalized individualism and its social and political consequences*. London, England: Sage.

Belek, B. (2018). Autism and the proficiency of social ineptitude: Probing the rules of "appropriate" behavior. *Ethos*, 46, 161–179.

Bellah, R. N., Madsen, R., Sullivan, W. M., Swidler, A., & Tipton, S. M. (1985). *Habits of the heart: Individualism and commitment in American life.* Berkeley: University of California Press.

Belmonte, M. K. (2008). Human, but more so: What the autistic brain tells us about the process of narrative. In M. Osteen (Ed.), *Autism and representation* (pp. 166–180). Abingdon-on-Thames, England: Routledge.

Biklen, D. (2005). *Autism and the myth of the person alone.* New York, NY: NYU Press.

Bishop-Fitzpatrick, L., Mazefsky, C., & Eack, S. (2018). The combined impact of social support and perceived stress on quality of life in adults with autism spectrum disorder and without intellectual disability. *Autism, 22,* 703–711.

Blaxill, M. (2004). What's going on? The question of time trends in autism. *Public Health Reports, 119,* 536–551.

Booth, R., & Happé, F. (2010). "Hunting with a knife and . . . fork": Examining central coherence in autism, attention deficit/hyperactivity disorder, and typical development with a linguistic task. *Journal of Experimental Child Psychology, 107,* 377–393.

Born, C. A. (2009). In the footsteps of the master: Confucian values in anime and manga. *ASIANetwork Exchange: A Journal for Asian Studies in the Liberal Arts, 17*(1), 39–53.

Brezis, R. S. (2015). Memory integration in the autobiographical narratives of individuals with autism. *Frontiers in Human Neuroscience, 9,* 76. https://doi.org/10.3389/fnhum.2015.00076

Brezis, R. S., Singhal, N., Daley, T., Barua, M., Piggot, J., Chollera, S., . . . Weisner, T. (2016). Self-and other-descriptions by individuals with autism spectrum disorder in Los Angeles and New Delhi: Bridging cross-cultural psychology and neurodiversity. *Culture and Brain, 4,* 113–133.

Broderick, A. A. (2010). Autism as enemy: Metaphor and cultural politics. In Z. Leonardo (Ed.), *Handbook of cultural politics and education* (pp. 237–268). Leiden, the Netherlands: Brill Sense.

Broderick, A. A., & Ne'eman, A. (2008). Autism as metaphor: Narrative and counternarrative. *International Journal of Inclusive Education, 12,* 459–476.

Brodwin, P. (2013). *Everyday ethics: Voices from the front line of community psychiatry.* Berkeley: University of California Press.

Brunsdon, V., & Happé, F. (2014). Exploring the "fractionation" of autism at the cognitive level. *Autism, 18,* 17–30.

Burd, L., Fisher, F., & Kerbeshian, J. (1987). A prevalence study of pervasive developmental disorders in North Dakota. *Journal of the American Academy of Child and Adolescent Psychiatry, 26,* 700–703.

Calabrese, J. D. (2013). *A different medicine: Postcolonial healing in the Native American Church.* Oxford, England: Oxford University Press.

Cascio, M. A. (2017). Operationalizing new biopolitical theory for anthropological inquiry. *Anthropological Quarterly, 90,* 193–224.

Cascio, M. A. (2018). What are we talking about when we talk about autism? In E. Fein & C. Rios (Eds.), *Autism in translation: An intercultural conversation on autism spectrum conditions* (pp. 251–259). New York, NY: Palgrave Macmillan.

Cascio, M. A., Costa Andrada, B., & Bezerra Jr., B. (2018). Psychiatric reform and autism services in Italy and Brazil. In E. Fein & C. Rios (Eds.), *Autism in translation: An intercultural conversation on autism spectrum conditions* (pp. 53–88). New York, NY: Palgrave Macmillan.

Castellani, P. J. (2005). *From snake pits to cash cows: Politics and public institutions in New York.* New York, NY: SUNY Press.

Center for Appropriate Dispute Resolution in Education. (2014). *IDEA special education due process complaints/hearing requests including expedited hearing requests.* Eugene, Oregon: Author.

Centers for Disease Control and Prevention (2019). Data and statistics on autism spectrum disorder. Available at cdc.gov.

Chapman, R. (n.d.). Intersectional neurodiversity: Reordering the differences. Available at https://intersectionalneurodiversity.wordpress.com

Charlton, B. (2013, May 22). Defining my dyslexia. *New York Times.* Available at https://www.nytimes.com

Charney, D. S., Barlow, D. H., Botteron, K., Cohen, J. D., Goldman, D., Gur, R. E., . . . Zalcman, S. J. (2002). Neuroscience research agenda to guide development of a pathophysiologically based classification system. In D. J. Kupfer, M. B. First, & D. A. Regier (Eds.), *A research agenda for DSM-V* (pp. 31–84). Washington, DC: American Psychiatric Association.

Clark, C. D. (2003). *In sickness and in play: Children coping with chronic illness.* Piscataway, NJ: Rutgers University Press.

Collins, F. (2012). The symphony inside your brain [Blog post]. Available at https://directorsblog.nih.gov

Constantino, J., & Todd, R. (2003). Autistic traits in the general population: A twin study. *Archives of General Psychiatry, 60,* 524–530.

Craig, F., Margari, F., Legrottaglie, A. R., Palumbi, R., De Giambattista, C., & Margari, L. (2016). A review of executive function deficits in autism spectrum disorder and attention-deficit/hyperactivity disorder. *Neuropsychiatric Disease and Treatment, 12,* 1191–1202.

Cure Autism Now. (2005). Kidnapped. Available at www.cureautismnow.org

Cuthbert, B. N. (2014). The RDoC framework: Facilitating transition from ICD/DSM to dimensional approaches that integrate neuroscience and psychopathology. *World Psychiatry, 13,* 28–35.

Czech, H. (2018). Hans Asperger, national socialism, and "race hygiene" in Nazi-era Vienna. *Molecular Autism, 9*(1), 29.

Dawson, G. (2009). *Introduction/Autism Speaks strategic plan.* Presented at the International Meeting for Autism Research, Chicago, IL.

Dawson, M., & Mottron, L. (2009). *Where autistics excel: Compiling an inventory of autistic cognitive strengths.* Poster presented at the International Meeting for Autism Research, Chicago, IL.

de Jonge, M. V., Kemner, C., & van Engeland, H. (2006). Superior disembedding performance of high-functioning individuals with autism spectrum disorders and their parents: The need for subtle measures. *Journal of Autism and Developmental Disorders, 36,* 677–683.

de Jonge, M., Parr, J., Rutter, M., Wallace, S., Kemner, C., Bailey, A., . . . Pickles, A. (2015). New interview and observation measures of the broader autism phenotype: Group differentiation. *Journal of Autism and Developmental Disorders, 45,* 893–901.

Dean, M., Harwood, R., & Kasari, C. (2017). The art of camouflage: Gender differences in the social behaviors of girls and boys with autism spectrum disorder. *Autism, 21,* 678–689.

Department of Health and Human Services. (n.d.). Standards for privacy of individually identifiable health information; final rule. Available at www.hhs.gov

Diament, M. (2016, October 14). Autism Speaks no longer seeking cure. *Disability Scoop.* Available at https://www.disabilityscoop.com

Dumit, J. (2004). *Picturing personhood: Brain scans and biomedical identity.* Princeton, NJ: Princeton University Press.

Dunn, W., Saiter, J., & Rinner, L. (2002) Asperger Syndrome and sensory processing: A conceptual model and guidance for intervention planning. *Focus on Autism and Other Developmental Disabilities, 17,* 172–185.

Duvekot, J., van der Ende, J., Verhulst, F. C., Slappendel, G., van Daalen, E., Maras, A., & Greaves-Lord, K. (2017). Factors influencing the probability of a diagnosis of autism spectrum disorder in girls versus boys. *Autism, 21,* 646–658.

Edelson. S. (n.d.) Autism research: standing on the shoulders of giants. Available at autism.org.

Eide, B., & Eide, F. (2012). *The dyslexic advantage: Unlocking the hidden potential of the dyslexic brain.* New York, NY: Penguin.

Ewing, E. L. (2018). *Ghosts in the schoolyard: Racism and school closings on Chicago's South Side.* Chicago, IL: University of Chicago Press.

Eyal, G., Hart, B., Oncluer, E., Oren, N., & Rossi, N. (2010). *The autism matrix: The social origins of the autism epidemic.* New York, NY: Polity.

Fein, E. (2015). Making meaningful worlds: Roleplaying subcultures and the autism spectrum. *Culture, Medicine, and Psychiatry, 39,* 299–321.

Fitzgerald, D. (2017). *Tracing autism: Uncertainty, ambiguity, and the affective labor of neuroscience.* Seattle: University of Washington Press.

Fombonne, E. (2005). The changing epidemiology of autism. *Journal of Applied Research in Intellectual Disabilities, 18,* 281–294.

Fombonne, E., & Tidmarsh, L. (2003). Epidemiologic data on Asperger disorder. *Child and Adolescent Psychiatric Clinics, 12*(1), 15–21.

Frith, U. (1989). Autism: Explaining the Enigma. Oxford: Blackwell.

Frith, U. (2012). Why we need cognitive explanations of autism. *The Quarterly Journal of Experimental Psychology, 65,* 2073–2092.

Gaiman, N. (1989). *Preludes and nocturnes* (Vol. 1). New York, NY: Vertigo.

Gee, J. (2005). Semiotic social spaces and affinity spaces. In D. Baron and K. Tusting (Eds.). Beyond Communities of Practice: Language, Power and Social Context. Cambridge: Cambridge University Press.

Geertz, C. (2000). *The interpretation of cultures: Selected essays (2000 ed.).* New York, NY: Basic Books.

Gernsbacher, M. A., Dawson, M., & Hill Goldsmith, H. (2005). Three reasons not to believe in an autism epidemic. *Current Directions in Psychological Science, 14,* 55–58.

Gernsbacher, M. A., Dawson, M., & Mottron, L. (2006). Autism: common, heritable, but not harmful. *Behavioral and Brain Sciences, 29,* 413–414.

Gillespie-Lynch, K., Kapp, S. K., Brooks, P. J., Pickens, J., & Schwartzman, B. (2017, March 28). Whose expertise is it? Evidence for autistic adults as critical autism experts. *Frontiers in Psychology, 8,* 438. https://doi.org/10.3389/fpsyg.2017.00438

Glidden, D., Bouman, W. P., Jones, B. A., & Arcelus, J. (2016). Gender dysphoria and autism spectrum disorder: A systematic review of the literature. *Sexual Medicine Reviews, 4*(1), 3–14.

Good, B. J., Herrera, H., Good, M. J. D., & Cooper, J. (1985). Reflexivity, countertransference and clinical ethnography: A case from a psychiatric cultural consultation clinic. In R. Hahn & A. Gaines (Eds.), *Physicians of Western medicine* (pp. 193–221). Dordrecht, the Netherlands: Springer.

Gotham, K., Marvin, A. R., Taylor, J. L., Warren, Z., Anderson, C. M., Law, P. A., ... Lipkin, P. H. (2015). Characterizing the daily life, needs, and priorities of adults with autism spectrum disorder from Interactive Autism Network data. *Autism, 19,* 794–804.

Graby, S. (2015). Neurodiversity: Bridging the gap between the disabled people's movement and the mental health system survivors' movement. In H. Spandler, J. Anderson, & B. Spadey (Eds.), *Madness, distress and the politics of disablement* (pp. 231–44). Chicago, IL: Policy Press.

Gray, K. M., Keating, C. M., Taffe, J. R., Brereton, A. V., Einfeld, S. L., Reardon, T. C., & Tonge, B. J. (2014). Adult outcomes in autism: Community inclusion and living skills. *Journal of Autism and Developmental Disorders, 44,* 3006–3015.

Green, J., Gilchrist, A., Burton, D., & Cox, A. (2000). Social and psychiatric functioning in adolescents with Asperger syndrome compared with conduct disorder. *Journal of Autism and Developmental Disorders, 30,* 279–293.

Greene, R. (1998). *The explosive child: A new approach for understanding and parenting easily frustrated, chronically inflexible children.* New York, NY: Harper Collins.

Greene, R. [DrRossGreene]. (2010, September 10) *Kids do well if they can Ross Greene #1.* [Video file]. Available at https://www.youtube.com/watch?v=jvzQQDfAL-Q

Greene, R. (2012, March). *Kids do well if they can: Collaborative problem-solving for parents and professionals.* Presentation to Family Action Network, Winnetka, IL.

Greene, R. (n.d.). Bill of rights for behaviorally challenging kids. Available at https://www.livesinthebalance.org

Grinker, R. R. (2007). *Unstrange minds: Remapping the world of autism*. New York, NY: Basic Books.

Hacking, I. (1995). The looping effect of human kinds. In D. Sperber, D. Premack, & A. J. Premack (Eds.), *Causal cognition: A multi-disciplinary debate* (pp. 351–383) New York, NY: Clarendon Press.

Hacking, I. (2004). Between Michel Foucault and Erving Goffman: Between discourse in the abstract and face-to-face interaction. *Economy and Society, 33*, 277–302.

Hacking, I. (2007). Kinds of people: Moving targets. *Proceedings of the British Academy, 151*, 285–318. doi:10.5871/bacad/9780197264249.003.0010

Happé, F., & Frith, U. (2006) The weak coherence account: Detail-focused cognitive style in autism spectrum disorders. *Journal of Autism & Developmental Disorders, 36*, 5–25.

Happé, F., & Vital, P. (2009). What aspects of autism predispose to talent? *Philosophical Transactions of the Royal Society B, 364*(1522), 1369–1375.

Haueis, P., & Slaby, J. (2017). Connectomes as constitutively epistemic objects: Critical perspectives on modeling in current neuroanatomy. In T. Mahfoud, S. McLean, & N. Rose (Eds.), *Vital models: The making and use of models in the brain sciences.* (pp. 149–177). Cambridge, MA: Academic Press.

Hedley, D., Uljarević, M., Wilmot, M., Richdale, A., & Dissanayake, C. (2018). Understanding depression and thoughts of self-harm in autism: A potential mechanism involving loneliness. *Research in Autism Spectrum Disorders, 46*, 1–7.

Herbert, M. (2008) Learning from the autism catastrophe: Key leverage points. *Alternative Therapies in Health and Medicine 14*(6), 28–30.

Herdt, G. (1999). Clinical ethnography and sexual culture. *Annual Review of Sex Research, 10*(1), 100–119.

Hopper, K., Jost, J., Hay, T., Welber, S., & Haugland, G. (1997). Homelessness, severe mental illness, and the institutional circuit. *Psychiatric Services, 48*, 659–665.

Howlin, P. (2000). Outcome in adult life for more able individuals with autism or Asperger syndrome. *Autism, 4*, 63–83.

Howlin, P., & Moss, P. (2012). Adults with autism spectrum disorders. *The Canadian Journal of Psychiatry, 57*, 275–283.

Howlin, P., Moss, P., Savage, S., & Rutter, M. (2013). Social outcomes in mid- to later adulthood among individuals diagnosed with autism and average nonverbal IQ as children. *Journal of the American Academy of Child & Adolescent Psychiatry, 52*, 572–581.

Ingstad, B., & Whyte, S. R. (Eds.). (1995). *Disability and culture*. Berkeley: University of California Press.

Insel, T. R. (2010). Faulty circuits. *Scientific American, 302*(4), 44–51.

Insel, T. R. (2013, April 29) Transforming diagnosis [Blog post]. Available at https://www.nimh.nih.gov

Insel, T. R., & Quirion, R. (2005). Psychiatry as a clinical neuroscience discipline. Journal of the American Medical Association, 294(17), 2221-2224.

Jacobs, A. (2014, Winter). Fantasy and the buffered self. *The New Atlantis*, pp. 3–18.

Jenkins, H. (1992). *Textual poachers: Television fans & participatory culture*. New York, NY: Routledge.

Jenkins, J., & Barrett, R. (2004). Introduction. In J. Jenkins & R. Barrett (Eds.), *Schizophrenia, culture and subjectivity: the edge of experience* (pp 1–28). Cambridge, England: Cambridge University Press.

Jolliffe, T., & Baron-Cohen, S. (1997). Are people with autism and Asperger syndrome faster than normal on the Embedded Figures Test? *Journal of Child Psychology and Psychiatry, 38*, 527–534.

Kana, R., Libero, L., Hu, C., Deshpande, H., & Colburn, J. (2012). Functional brain networks and white matter underlying theory-of-mind in autism. *Social, Cognitive and Affective Neuroscience, 9*, 98–105

Kanner, L. (1943) Autistic disturbances of affective contact. *Nervous Child, 2*, 217–250

Kapp, S. K., Gillespie-Lynch, K., Sherman, L. E., & Hutman, T. (2013). Deficit, difference, or both? Autism and neurodiversity. *Developmental Psychology, 49*, 59–71.

Kaufman, S. R. (2010). Regarding the rise in autism: Vaccine safety doubt, conditions of inquiry, and the shape of freedom. *Ethos, 38*, 8–32.

Krahn, T., & Fenton, A. (2012). Funding priorities: Autism and the need for a more balanced research agenda in Canada. *Public Health Ethics, 5*, 296–310.

Kupfer, D. J., First, M. B., & Regier, D. A. (2002). Introduction. In D. J. Kupfer, M. B. First, & D. A. Regier (Eds.), *A research agenda for DSM-V* (pp. xv–xxii). Washington, DC: American Psychiatric Association.

Kupfer, D. J., & Regier, D. A. (2011). Neuroscience, clinical evidence, and the future of psychiatric classification in DSM-5. *American Journal of Psychiatry, 168*, 672–674.

Kurchak, S. (2018, February 22). Autistic license: Imagining a fuller spectrum of autism on TV. *Pacific Standard*. Accessed from https://psmag.com

Lai, M. C., Lombardo, M. V., Ruigrok, A. N., Chakrabarti, B., Auyeung, B., Szatmari, P., . . . MRC AIMS Consortium. (2017). Quantifying and exploring camouflaging in men and women with autism. *Autism, 21*, 690–702.

Lakoff. A. (2000). Adaptive will: The evolution of attention deficit disorder. *Journal of the History of the Behavioral Sciences, 36*, 149–169

Latour, B. (1993). *We have never been modern* (C. Porter, Trans.). Cambridge, MA: Harvard University Press.

Lehman, A. F., Alexopoulos, G., Goldman, H., Feste, D., & Üstün, B. (2002). Mental disorders and disability: Time to re-evaluate the relationship? In D. J. Kupfer, M. B. First, & D. A. Regier (Eds.), *A research agenda for DSM-V* (pp. 201–218). Washington, DC: American Psychiatric Association.

Lester, R. J. (2011). How do I code for black fingernail polish? Finding the missing adolescent in managed mental health care. *Ethos, 39*, 481–496.

Lima R. C., Feldman, C., Evans, C., & Block, P. (2018). Autism policy and advocacy in Brazil and the USA. In E. Fein & C. Rios (Eds.), *Autism in translation: An inter-*

cultural conversation on autism spectrum conditions (pp. 17–52). New York, NY: Palgrave Macmillan.

Logan, J. (2009). Dyslexic entrepreneurs: The incidence; their coping strategies and their business skills. *Dyslexia, 15,* 328–346.

Losh, M., & Capps, L. (2003). Narrative ability in high-functioning children with autism or Asperger's syndrome. *Journal of Autism and Developmental Disorders, 33,* 239–251.

Losh, M., Martin, G. E., Lee, M., Klusek, J., Sideris, J., Barron, S., & Wassink, T. (2017). Developmental markers of genetic liability to autism in parents: A longitudinal, multigenerational study. *Journal of Autism and Developmental Disorders, 47,* 834–845.

Luhrmann, T. M. (2000). *Of two minds: The growing disorder in American psychiatry.* New York, NY: Alfred A. Knopf.

Madrigal, S., & Winner, M. G. (2008). *Superflex: A superhero social thinking curriculum.* San Jose, CA: Think Social Publishing.

Magiati, I., Tay, X. W., & Howlin, P. (2014). Cognitive, language, social and behavioural outcomes in adults with autism spectrum disorders: A systematic review of longitudinal follow-up studies in adulthood. *Clinical Psychology Review, 34,* 73–86.

Malabou, C. (2008). *What should we do with our brains?* (S. Rand, Trans.). New York, NY: Fordham University Press.

Mandell, D., & Mandy, W. (2015). Should all young children be screened for autism spectrum disorder? *Autism, 19,* 895–896.

Markus, H. R., & Kitayama, S. (1991). Culture and the self: Implications for cognition, emotion and motivation. *Psychological Review, 98,* 224–253.

Marrow, J., & Luhrmann, T. M. (2012). The zone of social abandonment in cultural geography: on the street in the United States, inside the family in India. *Culture, Medicine, and Psychiatry, 36,* 493–513.

Martin, E. (1994). *Flexible bodies: The role of immunity in American culture from the days of polio to the age of AIDS.* Boston, MA: Beacon Press.

Martin, E. (2004). Talking back to neuro-reductionism. In H. Thomas & J. Ahmed (Eds.), *Cultural bodies: Ethnography and theory* (pp. 190–211). Malden, MA: Blackwell.

Marx, T. A., Hart, J. L., Nelson, L., Love, J., Baxter, C. M., Gartin, B., & Schaefer Whitby, P. J. (2014). Guiding IEP teams on meeting the least restrictive environment mandate. *Intervention in School and Clinic, 50*(1), 45–50.

Matson, J. L., & Kozlowski, A. M. (2011). The increasing prevalence of autism spectrum disorders. *Research in Autism Spectrum Disorders, 5,* 418–425.

May, R., & Yalom, I. (1989). Existential psychotherapy. In D. Wedding & R. Corsini (Eds.), *Current psychotherapies* (5th ed., pp. 262–292). Itasca, IL: F. E. Peacock.

Mayes, R., & Horwitz, A. V. (2005). DSM-III and the revolution in the classification of mental illness. *Journal of the History of the Behavioral Sciences, 41,* 249–267.

Mazurek, M. (2013). Loneliness, friendship, and well-being in adults with autism spectrum disorders. *Autism, 18,* 223–232.

McGuire, A. (2016). *War on autism: On the cultural logic of normative violence.* Ann Arbor: University of Michigan Press.

McWade, B., Milton, D., & Beresford, P. (2015). Mad studies and neurodiversity: A dialogue. *Disability & Society, 30,* 305–309.

Merleau-Ponty, M. (1965). *The phenomenology of perception.* London, England: Routledge.

Mol, A.-M. (2002). *The body multiple: Ontology in medical practice.* Durham, NC: Duke University Press.

Mottron, L., Dawson, M., Soulieres, I., Hubert, B., & Burack, J. (2006). Enhanced perceptual functioning in autism: An update, and eight principles of autistic perception. *Journal of Autism and Developmental Disorders, 36,* 27–43.

Murphy, M., Bolton, P. F., Pickles, A., Fombonne, E., Piven, J., & Rutter, M. (2000). Personality traits of the relatives of autistic probands. *Psychological Medicine, 30,* 1411–1424.

Murray, S. (2008). *Representing autism: Culture, narrative, fascination.* Oxford, England: Oxford University Press.

Myers, N. L. (2015). *Recovery's edge: An ethnography of mental health care and moral agency.* Nashville, TN: Vanderbilt University Press.

Myles, B. S. (2003). Behavioral forms of stress management for individuals with Asperger Syndrome. *Child and Adolescent Psychiatric Clinics of North America, 12*(1), 123–141.

Myles, B. S., & Southwick, J. (1999). *Asperger Syndrome and difficult moments: Practical solutions for tantrums, rage, and meltdowns.* Shawneee Mission, KS: Autism Asperger Publishing.

Nadesan, M. H. (2005). *Constructing autism: Unravelling the 'truth' and understanding the social.* London, England, and New York, NY: Routledge.

National Institutes of Mental Health. (2011). NIMH research domain criteria (RDoC), Draft 3.1: June. Available at www.nimh.nih.gov

Ochs, E., Kremer-Sadlik, T., Sirota, K. G., & Solomon, O. (2004). Autism and the social world: An anthropological perspective. *Discourse Studies, 6,* 147–183.

Ochs, E., & Solomon, O. (2008). Practical logic and autism. In C. Casey & R. Edgerton (Eds.) *A companion to psychological anthropology: Modernity and psychocultural change* (pp. 140–167). Hoboken, NJ: John Wiley & Sons.

Ochs, E., Solomon, O., & Sterponi, L. (2005). Limitations and transformations of habitus in child-directed communication. *Discourse Studies, 7,* 547–583.

Opar, A. (2019, April 24). In search of truce in the autism wars. *Spectrum.* Available at https://www.spectrumnews.org

Ortega, F. (2009). The cerebral subject and the challenge of neurodiversity. *BioSocieties, 4,* 425–445.

Ortega, F., & Vidal, F. (2011) *Neurocultures: glimpses into an expanding universe.* Frankfurt, Germany, and New York, NY: Peter Lang.

Ortega, F., & Vidal, F. (2007). Mapping the cerebral subject. *Reciis: Electronic Journal of Communication, Information and Innovation in Health, 2,* 255–259.

Orwell, G. (1945). *Animal farm*. London, England: Secker and Warburg.

Ozonoff, S., Pennington, B. F., & Rogers, S. J. (1991). Executive function deficits in high-functioning autistic individuals: Relationship to theory of mind. *Journal of Child Psychology & Psychiatry & Allied Disciplines, 32*, 1081–1105.

Ozonoff, S., Strayer, D. L., McMahon, W. M., & Filloux, F. (1994). Executive function abilities in autism and Tourette syndrome: An information processing approach. *Journal of Child Psychology and Psychiatry, 35*, 1015–1032.

Pellicano, E., Dinsmore, A., & Charman, T. (2014). What should autism research focus upon? Community views and priorities from the United Kingdom. *Autism, 18*, 756–770.

Pellicano, E., & Stears, M. (2011). Bridging autism, science and society: Moving toward an ethically informed approach to autism research. *Autism Research, 4*, 271–282.

Pennington, B. F. & Ozonoff, S. (1996). Executive functions and developmental psychopathology. *Journal of Child Psychology & Psychiatry & Allied Disciplines, 37*, 51–87.

Pitts-Taylor, V. (2010). The plastic brain: Neoliberalism and the neuronal self. *Health, 14*, 635–652.

Pitts-Taylor, V. (2016) *The brain's body: Neuroscience and corporeal politics*. Durham, NC: Duke University Press.

Prince-Hughes, D. (2004). *Songs of the gorilla nation: My journey through autism*. Athens: Swallow Press/University of Ohio Press.

Putnam, R. D. (2001). *Bowling alone: The collapse and revival of American community*. New York: Simon and Schuster.

Queerly Autistic. (2017, November 20). My autistic headcanons (and why I prefer them to most 'actually autistic' characters). Available at https://queerlyautistic.com

Rapp, R. (2000). *Testing women, testing the fetus: The social impact of amniocentesis in America*. New York, NY: Routledge.

Rapp, R., & Ginsburg, F. D. (2001). Enabling disability: Rewriting kinship, reimagining citizenship. *Public Culture, 13*, 533–556.

Reed, P., Giles, A., Gavin, M., Carter, N., & Osborne, L. (2016). Loneliness and social anxiety mediate the relationship between Autism Quotient and quality of life in university students. *Journal of Developmental and Physical Disabilities, 28*, 723–733.

Rees, T. (2010). Being neurologically human today: Life and science and adult cerebral plasticity (an ethical analysis). *American Ethnologist, 27*, 150–166.

Rees, T. (2016). *Plastic reason: An anthropology of brain science in embryogenetic terms*. Berkeley: University of California Press.

Regier, D. A. (2007). Dimensional approaches to psychiatric classification: Refining the research agenda for DSM-V: An introduction. *International Journal of Methods in Psychiatric Research, 16*(Suppl. 1), S1–S5.

Research and Training Center on Independent Living, University of Kansas. (2008). *Guidelines for reporting and writing about people with disabilities* (7th ed.). Lawrence, KS: Author.

Ritvo, E., Freedman, B. J., Pingree, C., Mason-Brothers, A., Jorde, L., Jenson, W. M., . . . Ritvo, A. (1989). The UCLA-University of Utah Epidemiologic Survey of Autism: Prevalence. *American Journal of Psychiatry, 146*, 194–199.

Robertson, S. M. (2010). Neurodiversity, quality of life, and autistic adults: Shifting research and professional focuses onto real-life challenges. *Disability Studies Quarterly, 30*(1). http://dx.doi.org/10.18061/dsq.v30i1.1069

Robinson, S., Goddard, L., Dritschel, B., Wisley, M., & Howlin, P. (2009) Executive functions in children with autism spectrum disorders. *Brain and Cognition, 71,* 362–368.

Romoser, M. (2000). Malemployment in autism. *Focus on Autism and Other Developmental Disabilities, 15,* 246–247.

Rose, N. (2003). Neurochemical selves. *Society, 41*(1), 46–59.

Rose, N. (2007). *The politics of life itself: Biomedicine, power, and subjectivity in the twenty-first century.* Princeton, NJ: Princeton University Press.

Rose, N., & Abi-Rached, J. M. (2013). *Neuro: The new brain sciences and the management of the mind.* Princeton, NJ: Princeton University Press.

Rosenberg, C. E. (2002). The tyranny of diagnosis: Specific entities and individual experience. *The Milbank Quarterly, 80,* 237–260.

Rosenberg, C. E. (2007). *Our present complaint: American medicine, then and now.* Baltimore, MD: Johns Hopkins University Press.

Roux, A. M., Shattuck, P. T., Cooper, B. P., Anderson, K. A., Wagner, M., & Narendorf, S. C. (2013). Postsecondary employment experiences among young adults with an autism spectrum disorder. *Journal of the American Academy of Child and Adolescent Psychiatry, 52,* 931–939.

Roux, A. M., Shattuck, P. T., Rast, J. E., Rava, J. A., & Anderson, K. A. (2015). *National autism indicators report: Transition into young adulthood.* Philadelphia, PA: Life Course Outcomes Research Program, AJ Drexel Autism Institute, Drexel University.

Satel, S., Marshall, J., Aslinger, E., & Lilienfeld, S. O. (2017). Neurohype: A field guide to exaggerated brain-based claims. In L. Syd, M. Johnson, & K. Rommelfanger (Eds.), *The Routledge handbook of neuroethics* (pp. 261–281). New York, NY: Routledge.

Schultz, K. (2017, March 29). A roundup of posts against Autism Speaks [Blog post]. Accessed from www.medium.com

Sheffer, E. (2018). *Asperger's children: The origins of autism in Nazi Vienna.* New York, NY: W. W. Norton.

Shweder, R. A. (2003). *Why do men barbecue?: Recipes for cultural psychology.* Cambridge, MA: Harvard University Press.

Silberman, S. (2015). *Neurotribes: The legacy of autism and the future of neurodiversity.* New York, NY: Penguin.

Silverman, C. (2012). *Understanding autism: Parents, doctors, and the history of a disorder.* Princeton, NJ: Princeton University Press.

Sinclair, J. (1993). Don't mourn for us. *Our Voice, 1*(3). Available at www.autreat.com

Singh, J. (2015). *Multiple autisms: Spectrums of advocacy and genomic science.* Minneapolis: University of Minnesota Press.

Singh, J., Illes, J., Lazzeroni, L., & Hallmayer, J. (2009). Trends in US autism research funding. *Journal of Autism and Developmental Disorders, 39,* 788–795.

Solomon, O. (2004). Narrative introductions: Discourse competence of children with autistic spectrum disorders. *Discourse Studies, 6*, 253–276.

Solomon, O. (2008). Language, autism and childhood: An ethnographic perspective. *Annual Review of Applied Linguistics, 28*, 150–169.

Solomon, O. (2010). Sense and the senses: Anthropology and the study of autism. *Annual Review of Anthropology, 39*, 241–259.

Speare, E. (1958). *The witch of blackbird pond.* Boston, MA: Houghton Mifflin.

Spiegel, A. (2005, January 3). The dictionary of disorder. *The New Yorker*, pp. 56–63.

Strauss, C. (2005). Analyzing discourse for cultural complexity. In N. Quinn (Ed.), *Finding culture in talk: A collection of methods* (pp. 203–243). New York, NY: Palgrave Macmillan.

Stevenson, J. L., Harp, B., & Gernsbacher, M. A. (2011). Infantilizing autism. *Disability Studies Quarterly, 31*(3). http://dx.doi.org/10.18061/dsq.v31i3.1675

Sucksmith, E., Roth, I., & Hoekstra, R. A. (2011). Autistic traits below the clinical threshold: Re-examining the broader autism phenotype in the 21st century. *Neuropsychology Review, 21*, 360–389.

Tammet, D. (2006). *Born on a blue day: Inside the extraordinary mind of an autistic savant.* New York, NY: Free Press.

Taylor, C. (2007). A secular age. Cambridge, MA: Harvard University Press.

Taylor, C. (2008). Buffered and porous selves. The Immanent Frame. Available at tif.ssrc.org.

Understood.org. (n.d.). Least restrictive environment (LRE): What you need to know. Available at understood.org.

van Schalkwyk, G. I., Klingensmith, K., & Volkmar, F. R. (2015). Gender identity and autism spectrum disorders. *The Yale Journal of Biology and Medicine, 88*(1), 81–83.

Vanegas, S., & Davidson, D. (2015). Investigating distinct and related contributions of weak central coherence, executive dysfunction, and systemizing theories to the cognitive profiles of children with autism spectrum disorders and typically developing children. *Research in Autism Spectrum Disorders, 11*, 77–92.

Varenne, H., & McDermott, R. (1998). *Successful failure: The school America builds.* Boulder, CO: Perseus Book Group.

Venton, D. (2011, September 20). Q&A: The unappreciated benefits of dyslexia. *Wired.* Available at www.wired.com

Verhoeff, B. (2012). What is this thing called autism? A critical analysis of the tenacious search for autism's essence. *BioSocieties, 7*, 410–432.

Vidal, F. (2009). Brainhood: Anthropological figure of modernity. *History of the Human Sciences, 22*(5), 5–36.

Vidal, F., & Ortega, F. (2017). *Being brains: Making the cerebral subject.* New York, NY: Fordham Press.

Vital, P. M., Ronald, A., Wallace, G., & Happé, F. (2009). Relationship between special abilities and autistic-like traits in a large population-based sample of 8-year-olds. *Journal of Child Psychology and Psychiatry, 50*, 1093–1101.

Walker, N. (2013, August 16). Throw away the master's tools: Liberating ourselves from the pathology paradigm. *Neurocosmopolitanism.* Available at http://neurocosmo-politanism.com

Walker, N. (2014, September 27). Neurodiversity: Some basic terms and definitions. *Neurocosmopolitanism.* Available at http://neurocosmopolitanism.com

Weiner, T. (2011). The (un)managed self: Paradoxical forms of agency in self-management of bipolar disorder. *Culture, Medicine, and Psychiatry, 35,* 448–483.

Wheelwright, S., Auyeung, B., Allison, C., & Baron-Cohen, S. (2010). Defining the broader, medium and narrow autism phenotype among parents using the Autism Spectrum Quotient (AQ). *Molecular Autism, 1*(1), 10–19.

Whiteley, P., Todd, L., Carr, K., & Shattock, P. (2010). Gender ratios in autism, Asperger syndrome and autism spectrum disorder. *Autism Insights 2010*(2), 17–24.

Wilkinson, L. A. (2008). The gender gap in Asperger Syndrome: Where are the girls? *Teaching Exceptional Children Plus, 4*(4), Article 3. Available at https://files.eric. ed.gov/fulltext/EJ967482.pdf

Winner, M. G. (2015). Superflex, the team of Unthinkables, and the five step power plan. Available at www.socialthinking.com

Winner, M. G. (2018). Superflex: Helping kids become better social detectives, thinkers, and problem solvers. Available at www.socialthinking.com

Winner, M. G., & Crook, P. (2011). *Social fortune or social fate: A social thinking graphic novel map for social quest seekers.* San Jose, CA: Think Social Publishing.

World Health Organization. (2018, April 2). Autism spectrum disorders. Available at www.who.int

Wright, S., & Wright, B. (2014). A message from Suzanne and Bob Wright. Available at https://web.archive.org/

Yergeau, M. (2018). *Authoring autism: On rhetoric and neurological queerness.* Durham, NC: Duke University Press.

Yusuf, A., & Elsabbagh, M. (2015). At the cross-roads of participatory research and biomarker discovery in autism: The need for empirical data. *BMC Medical Ethics, 16*(1), 88.

INDEX

ABOUT THE AUTHOR

Elizabeth Fein is Assistant Professor in the Department of Psychology at Duquesne University. She holds a PhD from the University of Chicago Department of Comparative Human Development. She is a licensed psychologist in the state of Pennsylvania and the lead singer of Pittsburgh synthpop band Take Me With You.

Printed and bound by CPI Group (UK) Ltd, Croydon, CR0 4YY

27/10/2024

14580397-0004